DYSPNEA

Edited by
Donald A. Mahler, M.D.

DYSPNEA

Edited by

Donald A. Mahler, M.D.
Associate Professor of Medicine,
Dartmouth Medical School
Chief, Pulmonary Section,
Dartmouth-Hitchcock Medical Center
Hanover, New Hampshire

**Futura Publishing
Company, Inc.**
Mount Kisco, NY
1990

Library of Congress Cataloging-in-Publication Data

Dyspnea / edited by Donald A. Mahler.
    p. cm.
    Includes bibliographical references.
    ISBN 0-87993-361-5
    1. Dyspnea. I. Mahler, Donald A.
    [DNLM: 1. Dyspnea. WF 143 D998]
RC776.D9D97 1990
616.2—dc20
DNLM/DLC
for Library of Congress   90-3183
                                                                  CIP

Copyright © 1990
Futura Publishing Company, Inc.

Published by
Futura Publishing Company, Inc.
2 Bedford Ridge Road
P.O. Box 330
Mount Kisco, New York 10549

L.C. No.: 90-3183
ISBN No.: 0-87993-361-5

Printed in the United States of America

Dedicated to

my wife, Arlene,
my children, Jodi, Bethany, Ryan, and Brian,
and my parents, Milton and Esther,
*   with love and appreciation.*

Contributors

E. J. Moran Campbell, M.D. Professor of Medicine, Department of Medicine, Ambrose Cardiorespiratory Unit, McMaster University Medical Center, Hamilton, Ontario, Canada

Andrew Harver, Ph.D. Research Assistant Professor, Department of Psychology, State University of New York at Stony Brook, Stony Brook, New York

Susan Janson-Bjerklie, R.N., D.N.Sc. Associate Professor, School of Nursing, Department of Physiological Nursing, University of California, San Francisco, San Francisco, California

Kieran J. Killian, M.D., F.R.C.P.[C] Associate Professor of Medicine, Department of Medicine, Ambrose Cardiorespiratory Unit, McMaster University Medical Center, Hamilton, Ontario, Canada

Virginia Kohlman-Carrieri, R.N., D.N.Sc. Associate Professor, School of Nursing, Department of Physiological Nursing, University of California, San Francisco, San Francisco, California

Andrew L. Ries, M.D. Associate Professor of Medicine, Pulmonary and Critical Care Medicine, Department of Medicine, University of California Medical Center, San Diego, California

Foreword

At the top of any list of morbid complaints, shortness of breath lies not far below pain. In comparison with pain, dyspnea causes more anxiety and is less easily managed. It is certainly less well understood. Like all symptoms, dyspnea is a private phenomenon and inaccessible through the traditional techniques of physiology. It has been easier to list the causes than to discover the mechanisms. That is why the earliest attempts to study dyspnea took refuge in conducting further experiments on the control of breathing, because that was familiar territory and it was presumed to be somehow related to the subject at hand. It is not surprising that the results were more interesting than edifying. Scarcely thirty years ago, respiratory physiologists awoke to the fact that sensory physiology needs to be coupled with the psychology of perception if a true understanding is to be achieved. The era of respiratory psychophysics thus began, and a voluminous literature has resulted. And still, the goal remains elusive. A wealth of new information on the detection of elastic or resistive loads, volume and pressure estimation, and differences in scaling between healthy and diseased subjects has helped to complete our understanding of how conscious and automatic factors combine in the workings of the respiratory system, but it is debatable whether the mechanism(s) of dyspnea have been elucidated. Fortunately, the field is alive with good hypotheses, and clever investigators are designing experiments to refute them, but sometimes the fundamental problems appear to be philosophical as much as psychophysiological. At the start, language can be a hindrance, and words like fatigue and effort are lacking in precision; then, there is the problem of deciding whether some ordinary (and not unpleasant) respiratory sensation will, if sufficiently intense, cross some "threshold" and become dyspnea; and, most troublesome, the absence of an absolute reference standard for any sensory perception lays a notorious trap for the unwary.

The problem with a growing stimulus creating one sensory modality that leads to another (viz., dyspnea) without a change of mechanism remains debatable. This might be called the continuum assumption and a comparison with pain is illustrative of its potential fallacy. A light pinch excites touch, a moderate one pressure, but a hard pinch produces pain because pain receptors are excited at that stage, not because touch receptors were excessively stimulated. Similarly, mild heat is felt as warmth, intense heat as pain; thermal receptors first, pain receptors next. So, the stimulus may follow a continuous process, but the mechanism of the sensation it produces changes abruptly at some point. If there were a well defined "dyspnea receptor," our concept of the system would be much simplified. So far, there is no agreement regarding the existence of "dyspnea receptors," and, given the diverse causes of dyspnea, there may not be a single mechanism. It must be admitted: the symptom is complex.

Whether or not the absence of a standard in psychophysics is a serious handicap depends on the kind of information being sought, but it is almost always frustrating for a physiologist and his intuition is sometimes misleading. The temptation to assign some meaning to a non-zero response intercept on a stimulus response plot of a sensory experience is a seductive one, and even at its beginnings, that eccentric, ingenious pioneer of psychophysics, Fechner, saw the difficulty and formulated a theory that envisioned a finite quantity of sensations at the threshold of consciousness. The theory included a linking of an "inner psychophysics" with an "outer psychophysics" which joined a physical stimulus in the external world with the body (receptor physiology) and thence to conscious sensation by creating a kind of "internal energy," and this latter could be quantified by direct reference to the size of the external stimulus. There is an easy plausibility to an operation of this kind, but the system does not work that way. The central nervous processing of sensory information is more in the manner of a comparator whose bias is adjusted according to circumstance (hence, no fixed standard of reference), making states of mind, like attention, determinant. With such a moving yardstick, certain kinds of deduction are impossible, but the power of psychophysics is in no way diminished so long as the information it conveys is not overinterpreted.

Perusal of textbooks quickly reveals that discussions of dyspnea are still largely devoted to listing clinical causes. Several reviews examine current knowledge of (hypothetical) mechanism, but there are few monographs devoted to the subject of dyspnea, and none that treats the psychophysics of respiratory sensation and its relevant information for understanding dyspnea. Quantitative analysis of dyspnea is relatively new, and a summary now is timely, important, and useful. The editor and contributors of this volume have been close students of the subject, and they have provided a thoughtful assemblage of current knowledge together with practical applications helpful for the practitioner.

S. Marsh Tenney, M.D.
Nathan Smith Professor of Physiology
Dartmouth Medical School
Department of Physiology
Hanover, New Hampshire

Preface

Dyspnea is a symptom experienced by an individual as a distressing signal related to breathing. The affected person usually seeks medical evaluation when dyspnea interferes with his/her ability to perform certain daily activities. The physician tries to interpret the complaint in order to diagnose the cause and to reduce the severity of dyspnea. Although these encounters occur innumerous times throughout the day, dyspnea remains a perplexing problem for both the patient and the physician.

To begin with, there are basic limitations in communicating about respiratory sensations. Most people understand or have experienced difficulty in breathing, yet find it hard to describe. Furthermore, we do not understand the precise mechanisms which lead to dyspnea. Nevertheless, the physician is faced with diagnosing the disease as the most likely cause of dyspnea and then treating the condition. Because dyspnea is not usually measured, its severity may be unclear and the response to therapy may be uncertain.

The purpose of this book is to describe our current knowledge of the sensation of dyspnea. Our specific goals are to apply research findings to explain our understanding about the symptom and mechanisms of breathlessness; to describe and evaluate available instruments for measuring dyspnea; to review diagnostic approaches for acute, positional, and chronic dyspnea; and to present therapeutic strategies for reducing or alleviating the experience. Our collective efforts will only be successful if this book provides practical information which can be applied to the study, evaluation, and care of breathless individuals.

I wish to acknowledge my colleagues, E.J.M. Campbell, A. Harver, S. Janson-Bjerklie, K.J. Killian, V. Kohlman-Carrieri, and A.L. Ries, for their outstanding contributions to the various chapters in the book. Without their help, this book would not have been written. Also, I appreciate the thoughtful and critical comments of H.

Kotses (Chapter 1), A. Gift (Chapter 3), H.W. Parker and N. Yanofsky (Chapter 4), A.L. Ries (Chapter 5), G.L. Colice (Chapter 6), and B.R. Celli and N.S. Hill (Chapter 8). Finally, Mrs. Patti Holmes has been exceptional in preparing and revising chapters of this book.

Donald A. Mahler, M.D.

Contents

Chapter 1

The Symptom of Dyspnea

Andrew Harver and Donald A. Mahler

From *Dyspnea*, edited by Donald A. Mahler, M.D., © 1990, Futura Publishing Company, Inc., Mount Kisco, NY.

I. Introduction

Dyspnea is a medical term used to characterize the non-specific complaint of difficult breathing. It is the primary symptom of patients with a variety of disorders, especially those with respiratory disease. Many statistics convey the mortality and financial costs associated with respiratory disease,[1,2] but none convey the magnitude of either continuous or intermittent episodes of dyspnea. A statistical description of difficult breathing is unwarranted because there are no figures available for the symptom of dyspnea.

Until recent times, the study of dyspnea held little interest for researchers from clinical medicine, physiology, or psychology. In the 1960s, the first experiments designed to assess the ability of humans to detect resistive and elastic loads added to breathing were conducted by Campbell and colleagues.[3,4] In those experiments it was implicit that load detection and the experience of difficult, labored breathing likely were subserved by shared mechanisms.[5-7] Together with the introduction of direct scaling techniques to the conscious appreciation of respiratory sensations by Bakers and Tenney in 1970,[8] methodologies were put in place to examine these mechanisms as well as effects of mechanical and pharmacological manipulations on respiratory sensations.

During the past 10 years, there has been a surge of scientific interest in the measurement and neurophysiological mechanisms of dyspnea. A National Institutes of Health workshop on respiratory sensations was convened,[9] at least a dozen book chapters and review papers on the measurement and mechanisms of dyspnea were published,[7,10-21] and editorials concerned with the problem of breathlessness have appeared.[22-24] There has been also a noticeable increase in the application of sensory psychophysics to the study of respiratory sensations.[7,25,26]

This chapter is a review of the phenomenon of dyspnea, both as a symptom and as a sensory experience, focusing on clinical, physiological, and behavioral findings. Considerable attention is devoted to the methods of sensory psychophysics, results of psychophysical investigations of respiratory sensations, and the relationship between psychophysical outcomes and the symptom of dyspnea. Before examining these issues, three factors that complicate the discussion of dyspnea and relevant research concerned with the perception of physical symptoms will be addressed.

Most discussions on the topic of dyspnea include the terms breathlessness and shortness of breath interchangeably in order to characterize the subjective complaint of difficult, labored breathing. However, dyspnea may be conceived of as a class of experiences, and breathlessness, shortness of breath, and other similar physical sensations as orders or families of the experience. Such a taxonomic organization could possibly accomodate three factors that obscure the nature of a relatively common problem where little agreement is evident: (1) the various definitions of dyspnea, (2) the large and variable number of conditions in which dyspnea is a complaint, and (3) an array of discrete respiratory sensations used, in part, to model the symptom of dyspnea.

Dyspnea begs a precise definition. However, clinicians and researchers are prone to provide a formal definition of the subject.[14] A number of different definitions of dyspnea, or breathlessness, has been suggested, and examples are presented in Table 1. Dyspnea generally is considered separate from related ventilatory changes and physical sensations. It is not tachypnea, hyperventilation, or hyperpnea, and it is distinct from pain, fatigue, work, or effort,[12,27] but agreement on these issues is lacking also.[20] It may be wise to heed the advice of imposing a precise definition on the subject at this time.[28]

There is a large and varied number of conditions in which the symptom of dyspnea is a primary complaint, and the singular feature of these circumstances has yet to be elucidated. For example, a large number of patients with either cardiac or pulmonary disease–including those with congestive heart failure, chest trauma, obstructive airway disease, pulmonary fibrosis, and pulmonary vascular disease–complains of either acute or chronic episodes of dyspnea.[15,19,20] Attempts to distinguish between cardiac and pulmonary causes of dyspnea on pathophysiological bases have merit (see Chapters 4 and 6). But dyspnea occurs in many other conditions as well, including

Table 1. Definitions of Dyspnea Proposed by Various Authors

Definition	Reference #
1. The consciousness of the necessity for increased respiratory effort.	Meakins in 17
2. Unpleasant feeling of difficulty or inability to breathe based on the perception of real, threatened, or fantasied impairment of ventilation.	53
3. Pathological breathlessness.	10
4. Undue awareness of breathing or awareness of difficulty in breathing.	12
5. Difficult, uncomfortable, unpleasant breathing, but it is not painful.	15
6. A subjective expression of the perceptual intensity of stimuli that arise during or in association with the act of breathing.	25
7. Conscious awareness of outgoing motor command to the inspiratory muscles.	21
8. Quantitative non-threshold sensation of the motor effort required of the respiratory muscles.	18
9. Awareness of breathing that has become difficult or distressing.	14
10. Perception of reflexly mediated need for increased ventilation.	23
11. Increased effort in act of breathing.	24
12. Sensation of feeling breathless or experiencing air hunger.	20

neuromuscular disorders, skeletal deformities, psychogenic disturbances, hyperthyroidism, obesity, vigorous exercise, and pregnancy.[15,20,29] Dyspnea, apparent in so many conditions, would seem to invoke an invariant, multidimensional concept.

Most discussions of dyspnea have focused on the relevant experiences of the patient with lung disease. In the study of respiratory sensations, groups of discrete sensory experiences, evoked frequently by controlled, laboratory manipulations, have been catalogued and compared to the experience of dyspnea. For example, Comroe,[27] in summing up his observations of a 1965 symposium on breathlessness, concluded that there may be as many as five or six types or grades of breathlessness, including awareness of increased ventilation, shortness of breath, hindered breathing, suffocation, and the sensation at the breaking point of breath-holding. Guz[6] described four different types of respiratory sensations, including breath-holding sensations, irritation of the tracheobronchial tree, obstructed breathing, and the inability to get in enough air (induced by rebreathing carbon dioxide). Campbell and Guz[12] concluded that among the elemental sensations of chest tightness or irritation, excessive ventilation, excessive frequency of breathing, and difficulty in the act of breathing, the latter experience was consonant with classic dyspnea. More recently, the sense of tension or force, position or volume, displacement, and effort have been proposed to characterize fundamental respiratory sensations.[18,24,30] Elucidation of which of these discrete sensory experiences or combination of respiratory sensations delimits the symptom of dyspnea remains a formidable challenge.

The lack of a precise definition of dyspnea, the large and variable nature of the conditions in which it is a complaint, and the variety of discrete, conscious sensations available against which to evaluate dyspnea obscure the technical nature of the symptom of dyspnea. Numerous individual difference variables affect the perception of physical symptoms and serve to confound the subjective nature of dyspnea.

II. Perception of Physical Sensations and Symptoms

Recent scientific interest in the symptom of dyspnea parallels increasing scientific interest in the neurophysiological and psychological bases and mechanisms of internal sensations. A recent volume on neurophysiological mechanisms[31] addresses the various types of receptor activation, the transmission of visceral afferent signals in the central nervous system, and the functional organization of viscerosomatic convergence in the spinal cord and brain. A preoccupation with the role of visceral sensation in social behavior, including human emotion, and a constant struggle to develop appropriate scientific methods to assess objectively the perception of physiological sensations characterize a great deal of contemporary research in psychology.[32]

A. Historical Notes

The special senses—vision, audition, taste, smell, and touch—were classified centuries ago, and were known to Aristotle.[33] Until the late 1800s, however, philosophers and physiologists tended to ignore sensations arising from internal structures because sensations, regarded as the avenue by which the mind learns about things, normally must have an object, whereas sensations such as cramps, tickle, and hunger appear to have no object.[34]

The new science of psychology, which emerged from the synthesis of sense-physiology and the sensationistic psychology of the philosophers in the middle of the nineteenth century, continued to define sensation as the basic issue for study, including sensations elicited from within the body. Consistent with this history, virtually all motivational and behavioral theories within psychology have assumed that awareness of internal states affects behavior in some way.[35] Perhaps the most influential theoretical discussion of the role of physiological perception for behavior was generated by William James.[36] James suggested that when certain stimuli excited the visceral organs, the perception or "feeling" of the elicited bodily changes defined an emotion. The "object-simply-apprehended" became the "object-emotionally-felt." In more modern times, interest in the perception of physical sensations has evolved to include consideration of the processes and individual difference variables that affect the perception of physical symptoms.

B. Symptom Perception

A symptom is a perception, feeling, or belief about a state of the body.[37] Symptoms are used to guide and regulate behavior on a daily basis,[38] and the reporting of symptoms is highly adaptive and functional.[37] The perception of symptoms is a major link in the chain of illness behavior, the way persons monitor their bodies, define and interpret their sensations, take remedial action, and utilize the health-care system.[39] Health-care decisions are influenced by the visibility of symptoms, their frequency of occurrence, and the extent to which they are amenable to varying interpretive schemes.[39] The perception of symptoms is a factor that influences the mood, recovery, compliance, and functioning level of patients. In chronic conditions, for example, symptoms are readily available for monitoring the impact of treatment.[40]

The perception of symptoms is, in part, an attribution process, influenced by age, gender, and socioeconomic status.[37] Symptom attribution is the process through which persons identify and evaluate symptoms and make interpretations about their causes and implications. People actively identify and interpret symptoms based on beliefs.[35,41] Such beliefs are the result of past experiences with symptoms, and sociocultural information including the past experiences of others, social comparisons, and the mass media.[40] Modelling and other learning experiences during late childhood and adolescence also influence how adults perceive and react to somatic sensations.[42] The belief structures held or adopted by persons determine the type of information most likely attended to and encoded. With a given set of hypotheses, or schema, about the causes and implications of symptoms and illness, a person is more likely to encode schema-relevant information, i.e., evidence confirming expectations, than schema-irrelevant information.[41]

In addition to held beliefs, other individual difference variables that affect the perception of symptoms include sensitivity and reactions to changes in internal state, verbal acuity, tolerance to pain and discomfort, and psychological orientation. Although not exhaustive, these factors are relevant to many discussions of the perception of dyspnea. A summary of demographic, sociocultural, and individual difference variables that influence the perception of physical symptoms is provided in Table 2.

Table 2. Variables that Affect the Perception of Physical Symptoms

Demographic Variables
    Age
    Gender
    Socioeconomic status
Sociocultural Variables
    Personal history
    Social comparisons
    Mass media
    Social learning
Individual Difference Variables
    Beliefs
    Sensitivity and reactions to changes in internal state
    Verbal acuity
    Tolerance to pain and discomfort
    Psychological orientation

Individual sensitivity to changes in internal state varies widely, and considerable psychological literature exists concerned with the perception of physiological sensations.[32,37] Once the physiological signal is referenced accurately, however, reactions to the occurrence of symptoms may subsequently serve to modify the presence or level of the sensation and, accordingly, health-care decisions. The patient who recognizes increasing shortness of breath on exertion can easily avoid the sensory experience by using an elevator to reach a third floor office.

In general, patients find it extremely difficult to describe their physical sensations and vary considerably in terms of the accuracy or precision of their reports, particularly in the description of the causes of their symptoms.[16] However, because symptoms are private and subjective events, we depend on the verbal reports of individuals to characterize the nature of their experience. Intelligence, education, and verbal skills will affect the expression and idiosyncracies of patient descriptions.

The degree of impact of symptoms on a broad range of functions is related, in part, to the degree of tolerance to pain and discomfort. By collating behavioral, affective, and cognitive responses to pain, for example, three distinct subgroups or profiles of pain patients have been derived to direct treatment approaches in the management of various types of pain patients.[43] Patients are classified as dysfunctional, interpersonally distressed, or minimizers and adaptive copers, based, in part, on the perceived intensity of the pain experience and on the extent to which symptoms affect perceived levels of self-control.

Finally, psychological orientation, e.g., levels of mood, well-being, and distress, affects both a person's view of his or her health status and the interpretation of physical sensations. Bodily sensations such as pain, or dyspnea, may be reactivated under times of emotional stress, or may intensify when combined with an emotional interpretation to create a more diffuse sensory experience.[40,44]

III. Symptoms and Signs of Dyspnea

A symptom is any morbid phenomenon or departure from the normal in function, appearance, or sensation experienced by the patient and indicative of disease.[45] Symptoms are subjective, apparent only to the affected person. A sign, however, is any abnormality indicative of disease, detectable by another person and sometimes by the patient. A sign is an objective symptom of disease; a symptom is a subjective sign of disease.[45] Dyspnea is a symptom; tachypnea and wheezing are signs.

Some phenomenon, like fever, can be considered both a symptom and a sign of disease.[46] In this section is a review of the clinical, physiological, and behavioral symptoms and signs of dyspnea in patients with obstructive lung disease. The majority of investigations has focused on the sensory experiences of patients with obstructive airway disease in this context because it is a common medical disorder and dyspnea invariably is present.

A. Dyspnea: Sensation and Symptom

One area of agreement among clinicians and researchers is that dyspnea is a sensory experience, likely perceived in accordance with the same processes implicated in the perception of external stimuli. An awareness of a sensation—ventilatory increase, ventilatory difficulty, or ventilatory need[47]—is indicative of all definitions of dyspnea or breathlessness (Table 1). However, the mechanisms subserving the perception of dyspnea remain a matter of intensive scientific inquiry and debate (see Chapter 2). Many serious obstacles preclude understanding of the sensation, including homeostatic mechanisms. For example, it has been suggested for many years that the pattern of breathing is set to minimize the work of breathing.[48–50] Such patterns also may work to minimize respiratory sensations, including ventilatory discomfort.[51,52]

As a sensory experience, dyspnea is frequently compared to the sensation of pain. The experience of difficult, labored breathing is not painful in the usual sense of the word[53]; but dyspnea, like pain, is a multidimensional concept, varying along dimensions that are not intuitively obvious.[25] For example, pain varies not only in terms of its intensity, but also in terms of its qualitative attributes. Like pain, dyspnea is a symptom which frequently signals the need for medical attention. Unlike pain, however, dyspnea is not a generalized danger signal but is localized to the cardiopulmonary system.[44,54] Reactions to the sensation of pain, and to dyspnea, are affected by both motivational and emotional factors.

Verbal reports by patients of the sensation of dyspnea convey an extremely heterogenous set of experiences that can be differentially influenced by the underlying pathophysiology. Patients with dyspnea may simply complain of uncomfortable sensations arising from the chest or lungs, an inability to get in enough air, or chest tightness and congestion. The symptoms of patients with asthma are more variable than those of patients with chronic obstructive pulmonary disease (COPD).[16] Breathlessness in asthma is episodic and elicited by a variety of precipitants, but in chronic lung disease it is insidious and usually increases with physical exertion.[55] In addition, the sensory experience of dyspnea occurs in parallel with multiple, collateral sensations. The simultaneous presence of fatigue, numbness, headache, tingling, pain, exhaustion, muscular aching, apprehension, or dizziness further increases the range of symptom reports.[16,54,56]

The complexity of the pattern of symptoms experienced by patients with airflow obstruction has been characterized by Kinsman and his colleagues.[57–60] In one investigation, they considered the frequency of occurrence of a range of sensory experiences and symptoms present during periods of difficult breathing in 146 patients with COPD exhibiting moderate to severe levels of airway obstruction. The most commonly experienced symptoms were dyspnea (88%), fatigue (91%), sleep difficulties (74%), and congestion (chest tightness and wheezing; 79%). Three major types of symptom categories were derived from the interrelationships among these experiences: affective (depression, inability to enjoy others, anxiety); somatic (fatigue, congestion, numbness); and collateral (poor memory, sleep difficulties, alienation). In a second investigation, 176 patients with severe asthma rated the frequency of occurrence of 77 symptoms present during asthmatic episodes.[58,59] The most commonly reported symptoms were those of airway obstruction (hard to breathe, chest tightness, wheeze; 90%) and fatigue (78%). Three symptom clusters—mood, fatigue, and somatic—were derived to account for the interrelationships in reported symptoms. Episodes of difficult, labored breathing, in COPD and in asthma, are associated with, embedded in, and affected by a diffuse set of sensory experiences, as well as personal and social reactions.

Symptom discrimination, the first of a sequence of behaviors designed to attenuate or control attacks of bronchoconstriction, consists of both the awareness and appropriate interpretation of, as well as the appropriate response to, the changes in internal state that precede the onset of an asthmatic episode.[61,62] Unfortunately, many errors in the discrimination process can occur and these errors can result from a number of cognitive, behavioral, physiological, and environmental or physical events[63] (Table 3). Asthmatic patients unable to detect acute fluctuations in air flow could be at increased risk for more frequent and severe attacks of asthma.[61]

Pennebaker and colleagues[37,64] have emphasized that a careful evaluation of a patient's symptom reporting, in conjunction with physiological assessment, should be carried out in order to determine if the patient is aware of a specific phenomenological experience that is reliably related to the target symptom. Pennebaker[37] suggests further that the correlated perceived symptom is likely to be idiosyncratic, and that each patient may report a different, consistently reli-

---

Table 3. Classification of Errors in Symptom Discrimination

Lack of knowledge about:
  Precipitants of attacks
  Precipitant of a given attack

Misinterpretation or misperception of environmental/physical stimuli as
    precipitants

Failure to detect symptoms:
  Physiological failure
  Cognitive failure
  Contextual variables

Misidentification of physiological signs:
  Identification of sign as signal for attack when it is not
  Misidentification of respiratory change as not signaling attack when it
    does
  Misidentification of normal respiratory change as a signal for asthma

Failure in interpretation:
  Failure to understand meaning of physiological sign
  Failure to use physiological sign

Failure to initiate treatment:
  Lack of knowledge of what to do
  Failure to seek assistance

From Creer TL. Response: Self-management psychology and the treatment of childhood asthma. J Allergy Clin Immunol 1983; 72:607–610, with permission.

able correlate of the target symptom. With this approach, it may be easier to train patients to attend to their "naturally occurring" symptoms rather than to train them to make extremely difficult physiological discriminations. On the other hand, when patients are instructed to focus on their target symptoms, a change in the naturally occurring relationship between the underlying disorder and the corresponding symptom may result.

B. Clinical Presentations

The typical (non-asthmatic) patient who seeks medical help for dyspnea is a male between the fifth and sixth decade of life with a long history of cigarette smoking (20 pack-years or more) and/or chronic exposure to airborne irritants. Primary symptoms may include a history of chronic, productive cough, episodic wheezing, and various degrees of shortness of breath increasingly associated with exertion, e.g., climbing stairs and carrying packages.[54,65-67]

The clinical history serves to document the frequency, intensity, duration, and precipitants of the dyspneic episode. Knowledge about the history of onset, such as whether dyspnea occurs at night (paroxysmal dyspnea) while upright (platypnea) or recumbent (orthopnea), or worsens during acute infections, in the morning before secretions are cleared, or following large meals, is critical for understanding the problem and for developing therapeutic strategies. Information about how the disease has affected patient relationships, as well as its impact on occupational and recreational activities, supplements the clinical history.

The clinical examination may yield ample evidence to corroborate the patient's symptoms. Breathing may appear labored at rest or while talking; wheezing may be audible, and considerable use of the accessory muscles of respiration may be evident. Prolonged expiration through pursed lips, paradoxical retraction of the lower ribs on inspiration, postural adjustments, i.e., leaning forward with the elbows bent, and a barrel-shaped chest are frequent signs of a dyspneic patient with obstructive airway disease.[54,65,67,68] These and other physical signs of COPD are summarized in Table 4.

Table 4. Physical Signs in Chronic Obstructive Pulmonary Disease

EARLY:	Examination may be negative or show only: slight prolongation of forced expiration (which can be timed while auscultating over the trachea—normally 3 seconds or less) slight diminution of breath sounds at the apices or bases scattered rhonchi or wheezes, especially on expiration, often best heard over the hila anteriorly-the rhonchi often clear after cough
MODERATE:	Above signs are usually present and more pronounced, often with: decreased rib expansion use of accessory muscles of respiration retraction of the supraclavicular fossae in inspiration generalized hyperresonance decreased area of cardiac dullness diminished heart sounds at base increased anteroposterior distance of the chest
ADVANCED:	Examination usually shows the above findings to a greater degree and often shows: evidence of weight loss depression of the liver hyperpnea and tachycardia with mild exertion low and relatively immobile diaphragm contraction of abdominal muscles on inspiration inaudible heart sounds, except in the xiphoid area cyanosis
COR PULMONALE:	Increased pulmonic second sound and close splitting Right-sided diastolic gallop Left parasternal heave (right ventricular overactivity) Early systolic pulmonary ejection click, with or without systolic ejection murmur With failure: distended neck veins, functional tricuspid insufficiency, V-waves and hepatojugular reflux hepatomegaly peripheral edema

From American Lung Association. Chronic Obstructive Pulmonary Disease, 5th Edition. New York, American Lung Association, 1981; 64, with permission.

C. Physiological Function

Results of both pulmonary function and exercise tests are used not only to establish a diagnosis of lung disease but also to complement the clinical evaluation of the patient with dyspnea. While invaluable to the diagnosis of disease itself, the correspondence between physiological function and the intensity of physiological sensations is imperfect. On some occasions there appears to be little or no correlation between these two quantities.[62,69,70] For example, Rubinfeld and Pain[71] observed that some asthmatic patients report no symptoms despite marked levels of airway obstruction. Additional investigations confirm that the ability of an individual patient to perceive airway caliber varies widely.[72–74]

D. Behavioral Assessment

Behavioral scientists have largely ignored the condition of obstructive airway disease and the accompanying symptom of dyspnea.[75,76] Except for research concerned with smoking cessation and asthma self-management, few investigations have been conducted to explore the relationship between behavior and lung disease in terms of either its overt motor, physiological, or cognitive-verbal aspects.[75,76]

1. Psychometric Evaluation

Behavioral instruments used to evaluate patients with lung disease assess three, overlapping areas of functioning: general symptomatology and psychosocial functioning, psychological functioning, and neuropsychological functioning. Instruments that have been used to assess functioning in these areas are summarized in Table 5.

The evaluation of the patient with lung disease in terms of general health status, social adjustment, activities of daily living, mood, hobbies, and recreational activities has been accomplished with a number of instruments including the State-Trait Anxiety Inventory, the Beck Depression Inventory, the Sickness Impact Profile, the revised Symptom Checklist, the Profile of Mood States, and the Quality of Well-Being Scale.[77-82] In this line of research, interrelationships among quality of life, dyspnea, and pathophysiological state have been explored.[16,68,83–86] These and other similar investigations emphasize the frequently dramatic impact of lung disease on the quality of patients' lives and serve to identify specific content areas for improving the management of patients.

Table 5. Instruments Used to Evaluate the Relationship between Behavior and Lung Disease

Instrument	Comments	Reference #
Sickness Impact Profile	Impact of physical disability on daily activities.	79
Profile of Mood States	Self-report of affect.	81
Symptom Checklist (SCL-90)	Physical symptom checklist.	80
Quality of Well-Being	Comprehensive outcome measure of health status and life quality.	82
Minnesota Multiphasic Personality Inventory	Multidimensional assessment of personality characteristics.	91
State-Trait Anxiety Inventory	Self-report of anxiety.	77
Beck Depression Inventory	Self-report of depression.	78
Halstead-Reitan Neuropsychological Test Battery	Tests intelligence, attention, language, abstract reasoning, perceptual motor skills, sensation, motor activity, and memory.	97

Breathing and the perception of breathing sensations are substantially affected by emotions.[87] For example, anger and anxiety are associated with hyperventilation and the feeling that breathing is hard and fast; depression is associated with hypoventilation and the feeling that breathing is heavy and difficult.[88] Conversely, psychological factors are important in the self-rating of symptoms.[53] Breathlessness is a common somatic accompaniment of anxiety,[89] and a recent survey conducted in 600 healthy subjects demonstrated that those with more psychological symptoms (such as anger, anxiety, and depression) are more likely to report more respiratory symptoms (cough, phlegm, wheeze, dyspnea).[90]

Perhaps the most significant relationship between dyspnea and psychological functioning is the consistent observation that patients exhibit elevated scores on each of three subscales of the Minnesota Multiphasic Personality Inventory,[91] the most widely used and validated personality test in psychology. These subscales, referred to as the neurotic triad, assess depression (pessimism, hopelessness, slowing of action and thought), hypochondriasis (abnormal preoccupation with bodily functions), and hysteria (tendency to repress or deny the real presence of somatic complaints).[53,68,92,93] Anxiety also increases with increasing respiratory disability[94] and with increasing levels of dyspnea.[68] It is prudent to recognize, however, that many categories of patients, especially those with chronic physiological disorders, exhibit similar levels of dysfunction.

Subtle to moderate neuropsychological deficits that *potentially* reflect effects of subacute or chronic hypoxia have been observed in hypoxemic patients with COPD.[93,95] Results compiled from the Halstead-Reitan Neuropsychological Test Battery,[96,97] administered to patients participating in the Noctural Oxygen Therapy Trial (NOTT) and Intermittent Positive Pressure Breathing (IPPB) projects, revealed subtle to moderate levels of impairment in abstract reasoning, complex perceptual motor skills, concentration, problem solving, and short-term memory. However, intellectual functioning was preserved.[95] In the NOTT trial, 77% of the 203 patients tested exhibited clinically significant neuropsychological impairment. The observed level of neuropsychological impairment was associated with the severity of hypoxemia. Analyses of the combined NOTT and IPPB data pool, comprised of 302 patients and 99 controls, showed that more severely hypoxemic patients (mean $PaO_2 = 44$ mmHg) performed more poorly than those with either moderate (mean $PaO_2 = 54$ mmHg) or mild (mean $PaO_2 = 68$ mmHg) hypoxemia.[95]

2. Behavioral Consequences

Perhaps the most severe consequences of increasing levels of dyspnea are profound reductions in activity and emotional behavior. Physical activity or a strong emotion may initiate an unpleasant chain reaction, comprised of the interactions among fear, anxiety, and dyspnea, that may quickly accelerate.[44,88,93] Because of the fear of eliciting a dyspneic episode, patients may avoid the expression or experience of not only negative emotions, such as anger and anxiety, but also positive emotions, such as euphoria and general excitement.[44] Sleep disturbances, exaggerated respiratory complaints, and the losses of occupation, physical strength, and/or sexual potency are common consequences of increasing respiratory disability.[53,68,76,92,93]

3. Estimates of Sensation Magnitude

A large number of variables can be measured to estimate the magnitude of the sensation of dyspnea in both asthma and COPD. These include numbers of physician visits, the frequency and duration of hospital admissions, medication usage, activity levels, activity restriction, economic costs, daily peak flow recordings, verbal reports, and clinical dyspnea ratings.[61,69] However, none of these measures allows us to judge directly the subjective magnitude of the symptom of dyspnea. No test of pulmonary physiology or report of activity level provides for the conclusion that a patient's breathing is "twice as hard as normal;" no bronchodilator results in a "35% improvement in symptoms."

To predict what people will say when they try to give a quantitative description of their subjective impressions is to enter the domain of sensory psychophysics.[98] Sensory psychophysics is the investigation of the correspondence between the magnitude of stimulus properties as assessed by the instruments of physics and as assessed by the perceptual systems of people. Since 1970, over 100 studies have been published that describe the application of standard psychophysical scaling techniques to elucidate the intensity of respiratory sensations that arise during or in association with the act of breathing, including dyspnea.[7,22,25]

IV. Sensory Psychophysics

Excellent discussions of sensory psychophysics, including its history, may be found in the edited volume by Carterette and Friedman[99] and in various texts.[100–104]

A. Historical Aspects

The goal of sensory psychophysics involves seeking answers to two primary questions: (1) What is the ability of humans to detect changes in stimulus intensity? and (2) What is the ability of humans to judge changes in stimulus intensity? Answers to these psychophysical questions have been acquired through two complementary approaches to the scaling of sensory responses: indirect and direct. Although all psychophysical methods for collecting data are "direct," the dichotomy lies with respect to the way one constructs a sensation or response scale from empirical data.[100] In indirect scaling, measurements are derived from data on how well the observer can tell one stimulus from another; in direct scaling, the observer makes judgments of sensations that are then directly converted into measurements of sensory magnitude.

Classic or indirect psychophysical approaches are concerned primarily with the discriminability of stimuli and originated in the works of Weber and Fechner. In 1846, Weber reported that the "just noticeable difference," or JND, in intensity between two stimuli is a constant fraction of the intensity of the first stimulus.[105] Fechner, in 1860, used this formulation—subsequently known as Weber's law—to develop an empirical equation to describe the relationship between stimulus-sensation functions.[105] Fechner assumed that all JNDs were subjectively equal units and therefore proportional to the constant in Weber's law. By equilibrating JNDs with Weber's ratio, Fechner concluded that sensation grew as a function of the logarithm of the stimulus.[106] Accordingly, measurement of sensory magnitude comes about secondhand, as a function of the number of JND units above threshold.

Direct psychophysical approaches, however, have been derived primarily from the seminal contributions of Stevens.[98,104,107] Stevens[107] recollected that it all started from a friendly argument with a colleague, who said, "You seem to maintain that each loudness has a number and that if someone sounded a tone I should be able to tell him a number." In direct scaling, observers make judgments of sensation that are then transformed into measures of sensory magnitude, and functions are fit to stimulus-response pairs.[100] Through the use of direct scaling procedures, Stevens showed that physical intensity ratios yield corresponding sensation ratios according to a power function.

B. Detection of Stimulus Change

Detection tasks are designed to reveal absolute sensory (or stimulus) thresholds, difference thresholds, and terminal thresholds. The absolute sensory threshold (*reiz limen*) is the smallest amount of stimulus energy necessary to produce a sensation. The difference threshold (*difference limen*) is the amount of change in stimulus intensity required to produce a just noticeable difference (JND) in sensation intensity. The difference threshold is an ideal, statistical value computed from a number of observations, representing the central tendency of a response distribution.[108] The terminal threshold is the stimulus level beyond which further increases in intensity no longer produce alterations in sensory magnitude.

Three methods have been used to determine absolute and difference thresholds. Each consists of an experimental procedure and a mathematical treatment of the data. Each method has its advantages and disadvantages[108] and has been used to determine respiratory thresholds.[109]

1. Method of Constant Stimuli

The method of constant stimuli is the most versatile, accurate, and widely applicable procedure for determining sensory thresholds. Experimenters present a constant number of stimuli to subjects for a fixed number of presentations (possibly 50 to 200 times each). The number of stimulus intensities chosen (typically 5 to 10) are determined on preliminary trials and range from an undetectable stimulus to one that is always detected. These stimuli are presented repeatedly, and a psychometric function plotting the percentage of correct detections as a function of stimulus intensity is determined. Such a plot is displayed in Figure 1 which shows that the threshold value is interpolated as the stimulus intensity detected on 50% of the trials.

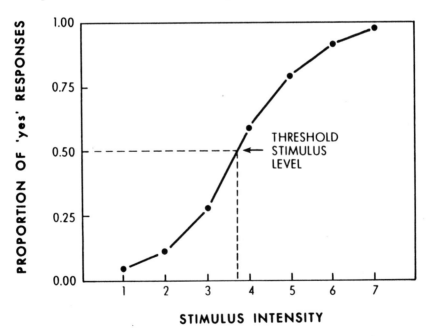

Figure 1: *Idealized psychometric function obtained with the Method of Constant Stimuli. (From Reed SD, Harver A, Katkin ES. Interoception. In: Cacioppo JT, Tassinary LG (eds). Principles of Psychophysiology: Physical, Social, and Inferential Elements. Cambridge, Cambridge University Press, in press, with permission of Cambridge University Press.)*

2. Method of Limits

In the method of limits (or method of minimal changes, or method of just noticeable differences), stimulus intensities are changed progressively by only a small amount until the boundary of sensation is reached. Stimulus intensities are changed in one direction only on separate ascending and descending trials. The transition point is determined using both ascending and descending sequences of stimulus presentations, which control for errors of habituation or perseverance (tendency to say "yes" in descending series) and errors of anticipation (tendency to say "yes" on ascending series). Variations of this technique include the staircase method, wherein stimulus intensity is controlled by the subject, and the forced-choice method, wherein the subject is forced to choose among several carefully specified observations, only one of which contains the stimulus.[103]

3. Method of Adjustment

The third procedure, the method of adjustment, is one of the oldest and most fundamental techniques, and the only method in which the subject has control over the stimulus. Active participation on the part of the subject in sensory threshold tasks may have intangible benefits.[108] In this method, the experimenter provides the subject with a standard stimulus and the subject adjusts a second, comparator stimulus until it seems comparable to the standard. A number of judgments are obtained from the subject, and their central tendency is taken as the stimulus value that is equivalent to the standard. The method of adjustment is also known as the method of reproduction, the method of average error, and the method of equivalent stimuli.

4. Weber's Law

As noted earlier, Weber's law, and its focus on the relationship between two stimulus values, provided the foundation for classic psychophysics.[100,105,106] Weber's law states that the intensity of a stimulus detected must be increased by a constant fraction of its original value in order to produce a minimum change in perceptual value. Mathematically, the relationship between the minimum change in stimulus intensity needed to produce a JND in perceptual value (ΔS) and the background sensory stimulus (S) is a constant (k), that is:

$$\Delta S / S = k$$

The greater the background sensory stimulus, the greater must be the change in stimulus strength in order for a subject to detect a change in stimulus intensity. Although robust in application, the Weber fraction increases rapidly near the extremes of both stimulus and terminal thresholds.[103]

By way of example, suppose an experiment is conducted to determine the difference threshold for luminance as a function of background luminosity. If the experiment starts with a room filled with 10 lit candles, and it is found that a subject can reliably detect the addition of one candle, the Weber fraction for luminance would be 1/10, or 0.10. Now suppose that the subject is brought into a room with a greater background sensory level, a room filled with 100 lit candles. According to Weber's law, 10 candles would need to be added to the room before the subject detected a JND in luminance. If true, the Weber fraction of 0.10 would be a constant, and would describe the relationship between the difference threshold and the background stimulus level for luminosity. Representative Weber fractions computed for a number of sensory continua are shown in Table 6.

Table 6. Representative Weber Fractions for Non-Respiratory and Respiratory Continua	
Continuum	Weber Fraction(ΔS/S)
Finger span	0.02
Electrical shock (skin)	0.03
Length of lines	0.04
Area (visual)	0.06
Heaviness	0.07
Brightness	0.08
Loudness (1,000 Hz tone)	0.10
Elastic loads	0.10–0.20
Taste (sweet)	0.17
Skin vibration (100-1,100 Hz)	0.20
Lung volume	0.20–0.30
Resistive loads	0.20–0.30
Smell (several substances)	0.24

Adapted from Baird JC, Noma E. Fundamentals of Scaling and Psychophysics. New York, J Wiley & Sons, 1978, with permission.

5. Signal Detection Theory

Sensory thresholds derived from classic psychophysical procedures do not take into account false alarms, i.e., the rate at which subjects indicate the presence of a stimulus when, in fact, none was presented. (Historically, such considerations were of little concern because of the use of highly trained experimental subjects.) To address this problem, as well as other problems introduced by response biases, signal detection theory (SDT) was developed. In signal detection tasks, the various factors that bias individual's reports are attenuated providing a relatively pure measure of discrimination.[110]

Response bias, and the variability it introduces in the determination of sensory thresholds, results from a host of non-sensory factors including the mood, personality, and motivation of the observer, and an oscillating background of sensorineural activity associated with random firing of the central nervous system.[110] One person may be strikingly willing to refrain from reporting the presence of a stimulus; another observer may strive to detect the smallest difference possible and accept a number of errors of commission. Consider the interpretation of a chest x-ray. When determining the presence of disease, the clinician may prefer a "hit" to a "miss," especially if the disease may be serious or contagious.[110]

In signal detection tasks, the subject is presented with a series of trials in which the stimulus signal is either present or absent. The subject may correctly identify the presence or absence of a signal (a hit), incorrectly identify a signal when, in fact, it was absent (false alarm), or miss the presence of a signal (a miss). Mathematical treatment of hit and false alarm proportions produces two estimates of the stimulus discrimination capabilities of a subject: (1) detection ability, and (2) the criterion used to judge the presence or absence of a stimulus. The first of these, d' ("d prime"), represents the observer's capability for making a discrimination; how well the observer is able to make correct judgements and avoid incorrect ones. The second, *beta*, provides an index of the subject's criterion for acting on information arising from the discrimination. Beta is thus an index of response bias, or riskiness of the observer in acting on the perceived discrimination; the extent to which the observer favors one hypothesis over another independent of the evidence he has been given. The effects of increased detection ability or increased response criterion on sensory thresholds is depicted in Figure 2. More details about com-

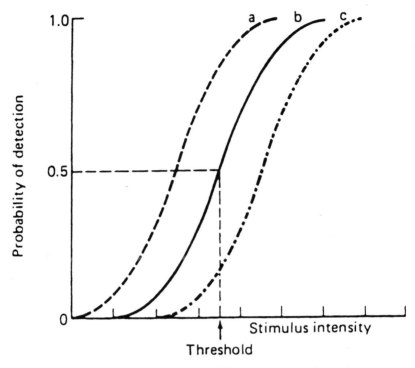

Figure 2: *Effects of either the detectability of the sensory system increasing or response criterion decreasing (curve a), or the converse (curve c), on an ideal sensory threshold curve (curve b). (From Martin J. Receptor physiology and submodality coding in the somatic sensory system. In: Kandel ER, Schwartz JH (eds). Principles of Neural Science, 2nd Edition. New York, Elsevier Science Publishing Co., Inc., 1985, with permission of Elsevier Science Publishing Co., Inc.)*

plex mathematical and theoretical issues in SDT may be obtained in Baird & Noma,[100] Gescheider,[103] and Swets.[110]

C. Direct Estimates of Stimulus Magnitude

Fechner, in 1860,[105] first suggested that sensory intensities could be measured and that the fundmental relationship between sensation magnitude and stimulus intensities was logarithmic. In other words, he argued, in part based on Weber's findings, sensation magnitude was equal to a constant plus the number of JNDs of stimulus energy above threshold. This analysis has subsequently been shown to be an incomplete assessment of sensation magnitude. For example, a doubling in loudness from 50 to 100 dB is subjectively much greater than only twice the physical increase; a 100 dB noise sounds 40 times as loud as a 50 dB noise!

Principles for direct magnitude scaling have been derived primarily from Stevens.[104,107] In direct scaling, observers make judgments of sensations that are then transformed into measurements of sensory magnitude. Stevens[107] developed the method of magnitude estimation to measure directly sensation magnitude in humans. In his analysis, equal stimulus ratios produced equal sensation ratios, and sensation magnitude grew as a power function of stimulus intensity. Stevens' power function equation has been shown to be invariant for many perceptual continua.[100] It suggests an underlying order in the perceptual transformation of the environment. The power function has been verified in hundreds of experiments for a wide range of perceptual systems.

There are two types of direct scaling tasks: category scaling and ratio scaling. In category scaling, the goal is to construct "equal sensation intervals" between stimuli of various intensities; in ratio scaling tasks, the goal is to construct "equal sensation ratios" between stimuli of various intensities.[100] The former tasks differ from the latter tasks in the following manner. In the construction of category scales, the subject works with a limited range and type of numbers to describe stimulus attributes; the extreme values of the scale are anchored by numerals supplied by the experimenter. In ratio tasks, there is no limit to either the range or type of the numbers an individual may use to estimate sensory attributes of the stimulus. Exponents derived from category tasks are smaller compared to those derived from ratio tasks.[100]

1. Category Scaling

In category estimation, the subject uses a limited range and type of number, for example one to ten; in assessing perceived magnitude, fractions are not permitted, nor are numbers outside the range.[100]

Stevens frequently admonished against the use of category scaling: "For the purposes of serious perceptual measurement, category methods should be shunned."[98] However, category scales, particularly Borg's category and category-ratio scales,[111,112] may have clinical utility.[24] They will be discussed later in the chapter.

2. Ratio Scaling

A ratio scale—a scale that possesses a unique zero—is the only one in which the concepts of "twice" or "ten times as much" have meaning.[100] The ratio methods permit subjects to use any numbers, including fractions, to judge perceived magnitude. In general, the subject is told to focus on ratio relationships among stimulus intensities. If one stimulus appears five times as intense as another, this judgment could be represented by the numbers 1 and 5, or 5 and 25. Several direct scaling techniques are used to assess the perceived magnitude of stimulus intensities.

a. Magnitude estimation and production: In magnitude estimation, the observer supplies a number to match the subjective magnitude of each of several stimulus levels. For example, an individual might rate the perceived magnitude of a series of auditory tones. In one version of the task, the experimenter provides a standard value (a modulus) for the stimulus of intermediate intensity; subsequent estimations by the observer are referred to that standard. In the other version, free or "open" ratio estimation, the subject provides an estimate of the stimulus level of intermediate intensity, and subsequent estimations are referred to this standard estimate. To minimize response bias, the latter version is generally preferred to the former.[104] When the estimations of several observers obtained with free ratio estimation are combined, the method of modulus equalization adjusts all the individual estimates to a common standard.[104]

In magnitude production, the subject is engaged in the inverse process: the observer is required to manipulate the intensity of a stimulus to match the subjective magnitude of a numerical value supplied by the experimenter. For example, an observer might produce a range of inspiratory volumes to match the subjective magnitude of numbers ranging between 5 and 160.

b. Cross-modality and magnitude matching: In the third type of ratio task, cross-modality matching, individuals manipulate the intensity of a stimulus in one modality, e.g., loudness, to match the perceived intensity of the magnitude of the stimulus of a different modality, e.g., light intensity. Cross-modality matching can be used to validate a given scale. For example, when responses from each modality are paired and plotted on logarithmic coordinates, the result is an "equal sensation function;" the slope of the best-fitting line between these corresponding units is given by the ratio of the two exponents obtained in separate magnitude estimation tasks. If a subject matches hand-grip strength (which has an exponent of 1.7) to loudness (which has an exponent of 0.3), the expected exponent of the resulting equal sensation function would be 1.7/0.3, or 5.1. Equal sensation functions according to Stevens[113] are presented in Figure 3.

In magnitude matching, or mixed-modality psychophysical scaling, magnitude estimations are obtained for two sets of stimuli from different modalities interspersed in the same test session.[114] Stimuli that are assigned the same average numerical value are taken as having the same apparent magnitude. A cross-modality matching func-

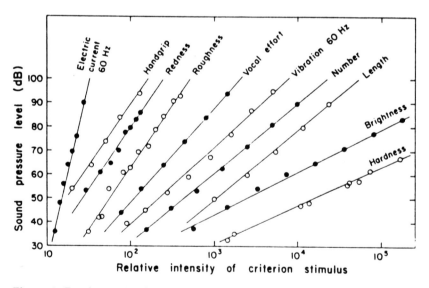

Figure 3: *Equal sensation functions determined by cross-modality matches between loudness and various criterion stimuli. (From Stevens SS. Matching functions between loudness and ten other continua. Percept Psychophys 1966; 1:5-8, with permission.)*

tion is obtained by plotting pairs of stimuli from the two modalities that produce the same magnitude estimation values. In this way, judgments can be normalized so that their absolute response values can be compared.[115] Magnitude matching may prove clinically useful. From a battery of cross-modality matching functions, specific sensory deficits may emerge when comparing groups of subjects.[114]

3. Stevens' Law

When one desires to evaluate the perceived magnitude of stimulus intensities, one turns to the construction of psychological magnitude functions, which plots the subject's attribution of the magnitude of the sensory experience against the corresponding objectively measured, physical magnitude of the stimulus. When plotted on linear, Cartesian coordinates, three functions can result to characterize the rate at which subjective magnitude rises as a function of changes in the magnitude of stimulus intensity. An example of each type is shown in Figure 4. Perceived magnitude may rise faster than stimulus magnitude, as is the case for electric shock; perceived magnitude may rise at the same rate as stimulus magnitude as for apparent length; or perceived magnitude may rise slower than stimulus magnitude, as in brightness perception.

Stevens[104,107] showed that physical intensity ratios yield corresponding sensation ratios according to a power function, where J is the sensory judgment of the stimulus, k is a scaling constant, I is the physical magnitude of the stimulus, and n is the relative sensitivity:

$$J = k\ I^n$$

This formulation (Stevens' law) states that the perceived magnitude of various sensory dimensions increases in proportion to stimulus intensity raised to a power. Stevens' law has been verified for a large range of perceptual continua, and has been examined under many stimulus conditions and with a variety of methodologies.

Regardless of the direct scaling method employed, the measure of correspondence between sensation intensity and stimulus magnitude is the slope of the regression line fitted between pairs of scores

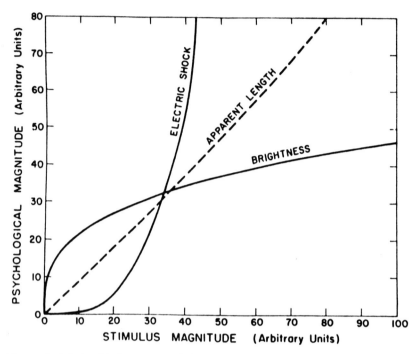

Figure 4: *Relationship between psychological magnitude and stimulus magnitude for three stimuli plotted in linear coordinates. (From Stevens SS. The psychophysics of sensory function. Am Sci 1960; 48:226-253, with permission.)*

obtained from two scales: numerical attributes of the sensation, and the corresponding initiating stimulus. The slope of the best-fitting line between these corresponding units, when plotted on logarithmic (base$_{10}$) coordinates, is taken as the measured exponent (n) in Stevens' law. Theoretically, the exponent provides information about the sensory processing of stimulus energies. When n = 1, changes in psychological magnitude correspond directly to changes in stimulus intensity. When n > 1, small ranges of physical stimuli are expanded into a wide range of psychological magnitudes; when n < 1, wide ranges of physical stimuli are judged with little corresponding change in psychological magnitude. Psychometric functions for various stimuli according to Stevens[104] are shown in Figure 5. Exponents for shock (3.6), heaviness (1.4), loudness (0.6), and brightness (0.33) are shown.

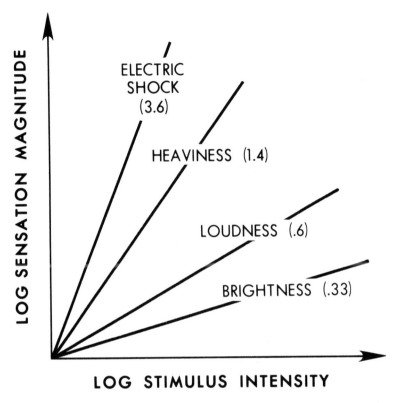

Figure 5: *Psychological magnitude functions for various sensory stimuli (logarithmic coordinates). (From Reed SD, Harver A, Katkin ES. Interoception. In: Cacioppo JT, Tassinary LG (eds). Principles of Psychophysiology: Physical, Social, and Inferential Elements. Cambridge, Cambridge University Press, in press, with permission of Cambridge University Press.)*

4. Response Bias and Validity of Measurement

There are no criteria for assessing the validity of psychological magnitude functions, although Stevens' law has undergone considerable theoretical scrutiny.[116,117] Recently, for example, a two-stage model of the basic components of the magnitude scaling task has been reviewed.[115] In that model, psychological magnitude functions are considered in light of both sensory and cognitive factors, as well as the complex interactions between both classes of factors.

No single psychophysical function characterizes a sensory attribute. The values of exponents are usually highly dependent on experimental conditions, for example, the spacing of stimuli and the size of the standard stimulus.[107] Many other variables in addition to stimulus intensity affect obtained psychological magnitude functions, including a subject's number behavior, the subject's conception of ratio relationships, instructions to attend to a single sensory aspect of the stimulus, and variations in biological quantities, especially sense-organ operating characteristics.[118] Sequential effects—the observation that responses on a particular trial tend to be positively correlated with responses on the previous trial—are one of a host of response biases that influence psychological judgments.[115]

At the other extreme, research has uncovered specific relationships between receptor physiology and sensory experiences to support the power law relationship. In many non-human species, actual recordings of neuroelectric activity from sensory receptors, nerve fibers, and neural complexes have been shown to follow power functions.[98,106,119] In the first experiment of this type conducted in humans, Borg and colleagues[120] demonstrated a "fundamental congruity" between neural activity recorded from the human chorda tympani in the middle ear (through which the gustatory fibers run) and the perceived intensity of citric acid and sucrose applied to the tongue. In addition, there are at least four sense modalities in which some particular aspect of the human cortical potential has been shown to follow a power function.[119]

5. Category-Ratio Scaling

An increasingly popular approach to examining the magnitude of physical sensations involves use of Borg's category and category-ratio scales.[111,112] In the late 1950s, Borg began his elegant analyses of the psychophysics of physical work (perceived exertion), and was later commended by Stevens himself for opening a new field of scientific inquiry. Perceived exertion—a multidimensional construct perhaps not unlike pain and dyspnea—results from the configuration of many perceptions and sensations arising from both local (e.g., strain in the muscles, peripheral proprioceptors) and central factors.[121]

In the 1960s, Borg observed that the relation between ratings of perceived exertion and heart rate was described by a positively accelerating function with an exponent of 1.6.[122] But Borg recognized also that these psychophysical (ratio) relations provided no index for evaluating subjective levels of sensation magnitude between individuals, and sought to develop simple rating methods to provide meaningful, interindividual comparisons. To this end, he designed a 21-grade category rating scale purposefully constructed to increase linearly with workload (heart rate),[112,122] and high correlations (range, 0.80–0.90) were obtained subsequently between ratings of perceived exertion and heart rate. The scale was modified to a 15-grade category scale (the "Borg scale" or rating of perceived exertion [RPE] scale) with values ranging between 6 and 20. At the same time, a range theory for both interindividual and intermodal comparisons evolved. Briefly, by calibrating perceptual intensities at maximal levels of stimulation, a frame of reference for equating perceptual responses within individual stimulus response ranges could be established.[111,121,123]

Category and ratio scales are non-linearly related.[100,104] Borg's subsequent efforts, therefore, concerned the development of a simple category scale that could be used not only to compare levels of perceived magnitude between subjects but also to describe ratio relationships between stimulus-sensation pairs. Knowing both the linear relationship between ratings of perceived exertion and physical work and the exponential relationship between these two quantities, Borg created a 20-grade scale in which the spacing of numerals accomodated the exponential relationship.[111] This scale was further simplified to the widely available 10-point category-ratio scale, and verbal expressions were placed strategically next to numerals to reflect "ratio" changes in perceived magnitude. In a sense, the multiplicative constants in Stevens' law were replaced with adverbs and adjectives.[124] A recent experiment provided evidence consistent with the range model for examining individual differences in perceived exertion during cycle ergometry using the category-ratio scale,[123] but such validation has yet to be established in a similar manner for dyspnea, or breathlessness.[24] It is unclear, for example, what physiological calibrator response might be used to equalize stimulus response ranges (cf. heart rate) in such an evaluation.

V. Respiratory Psychophysics

The first investigations of the ability of human subjects to detect just noticeable increases in either the resistive or elastic component to breathing were conducted by Campbell and his colleagues.[3,4] Bakers and Tenney[8] introduced direct scaling techniques to investigate the perception of respiratory pressures and volumes, and magnitude estimation was first applied to the perception of resistive and elastic loads fairly recently.[125] In 1986, Zechman and Wiley[26] published a "state of the art" review of the field of respiratory psychophysics that summarized about 50 experiments (including references to 12 abstracts) concerned with the quantification of respiratory sensations conducted through 1981. A comparable but more recent review would need to contend with results from a voluminous literature (over 100 published investigations) on the perception of respiratory volumes and pressures, ventilation, end-tidal carbon dioxide levels, and added loads to breathing, taking account effects of altered mechanical backgrounds, pharmacological manipulations, chest strapping, airway anesthesia, and constrained breathing patterns. Our review is necessarily limited. We focus only on selected observations of the ability of healthy subjects and patients with lung disease to detect and scale the magnitude of resistive and elastic loads.

Resistive loads alter normally present pulmonary pressure-flow relationships. Loads are constructed generally of units of porous material connected in series to provide linear increases in flow-resistance. From a clinical standpoint, resistive loads mimic the type of flow limitation experienced by patients with obstructive lung disease. Extrapulmonary load intensities are determined by passing air through the resistors at known flow rates and measuring the drop in pressure across the resistor that results ($cmH_2O/L/sec$). Elastic loads are produced by requiring individuals to breath from airtight containers of various sizes joined in parallel with tubing and normally vented to atmosphere. Breathing through an elastic circuit alters the pressure-volume relationships normally present, and mimics the type of volume restriction experienced by patients with restrictive lung disease. These loads are quantified by measuring the pressure within the container as known quantities of air are injected or withdrawn from the circuit. The ratio between the change in pressure for a given change in volume is a constant and describes the elastance of the container (cmH_2O/L). A schematic of both resistive and elastic loads is displayed in Figure 6.

In the laboratory, loads are presented to subjects for an entire breath or for only part of a breath, with or without warning. Following the presentation of a load, subjects are asked to decide whether a load was present (in discrimination tasks) or provide an estimate of the

Resistance Circuit

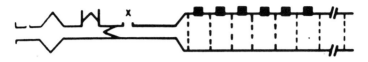

Elastance Circuit

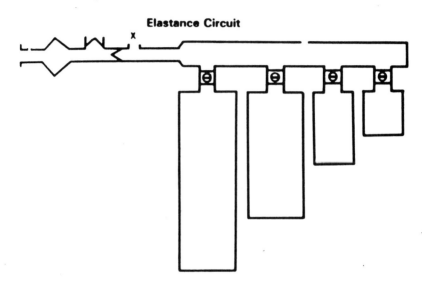

Figure 6: *Schematic of resistance and elastance breathing circuits. (From Killian KJ, Mahutte CK, Campbell EJM. Magnitude scaling of externally added loads to breathing. Am Rev Respir Dis 1981; 123:12-15, with permission.)*

magnitude of the sensation elicited by the load (in direct scaling tasks). In many direct scaling experiments, both the level of the added load and peak inspiratory pressure (an index of the tension produced by the respiratory muscles) are used as estimates of the initiating physical stimulus in separate power function calculations. The perceived magnitude of added loads is uniquely related to the force or effort exerted in overcoming the load, and indirectly related to load type.[126–129]

A. Detection Thresholds and Weber Fractions

The just noticeable increases in either the resistive or elastic component to breathing were assessed initially by Campbell and colleagues.[3,4] The elastic load detected 50% of the time was 2.47 cmH$_2$O/

L when the breathing pattern was unconstrained and 2.08 cmH_2O/L when the tidal volume was fixed to twice the average value. The just noticeable difference for resistive loads was 0.56 $cmH_2O/L/sec$ on one day, and 0.61 $cmH_2O/L/sec$ on repeated testing. More recent experiments have resulted in elastic and resistive load detection thresholds in the 1–1.5 cmH_2O/L and 0.5–1.0 $cmH_2O/L/sec$ range, respectively.[26,130] Compared to healthy subjects, elastic load difference thresholds are greater in patients with interstitial lung disease, and those for resistive loads are greater in patients with asthma and COPD.[26,130,131]

Difference thresholds for resistive loads bear a constant relation to the total background sensory stimulus, i.e., the sum of the resistance of the breathing circuit and intrinsic airway resistance. Bennett and colleagues[3] first demonstrated that the JND for resistive loads represented about a 25% increase in the resistive component to breathing. Subsequent experiments have confirmed that the Weber fraction for resistive loads (range, 0.2–0.3) is relatively constant for a wide range of background intensities and, as in other sense modalities, increases rapidly near stimulus threshold.[132,133] In patients with asthma exhibiting intrinsic increases in airways resistance, the JND for resistive loads is greater but the computed Weber fractions are comparable to those of non-asthmatics.[131,134] Similarly, the Weber fraction for elastic loads (range, 0.1–0.2) is comparable in normal subjects and in patients with interstitial lung disease.[130,135] However, both resistive load detection thresholds and the consequent Weber fractions are elevated in patients with COPD.[125,134] Weber ratios for a number of sensory continua were depicted in Table 6, including, for comparative purposes, results obtained from respiratory discrimination tasks.

Study of the non-sensory factors that affect resistive and elastic load detection ability—for example, anxiety[136,137]—has been recommended,[9] but only a few investigators have used signal detection tasks to evaluate sensitivity (d') and response bias (*beta*) in load discrimination. In one experiment, sensitivity to resistive loads presented throughout all of inspiration was equivalent to that for loads presented only during the initial, accelerating phase of inspiration.[138] In a second study, strapping the chest at full expiration prior to a resistive load detection task resulted in both detection sensitivity decreases and response bias increases compared to when the chest cage was unrestricted.[139] More recently, asthmatic subjects were found to be more sensitive than normal subjects to resistive loads applied either during inspiration or during expiration when sensitivity was expressed in relation to airway resistance.[140] These few paradigms reflect the contrast in perspective or focus between signal detection and classic approaches to load discrimination research.

B. Magnitude Scaling Exponents

From a relatively large number of investigations of the perceived magnitude of respiratory sensations, cohesive sets of exponents have accrued for different scaling tasks and for performance on these tasks in various subpopulations. For example, exponents for static respiratory efforts produced against a closed airway in young and old adults and in patients with COPD average about 1.5 to 1.7.[141-143] Exponents for the perceived magnitude of resistive loads added to inspiration in patients with COPD average about 0.5[144,145] and those in young adults are about 0.8.[52,127] In a number of experiments, the exponent for inspired lung volume has averaged about 1.2.[146] Representative exponents for several respiratory sensations are presented in Table 7 along with representative exponents for other sensory continua for comparative purposes.

A particularly relevant issue for the present discussion surrounding the direct scaling of resistive and elastic loads concerns the results of comparisons made among exponents computed for healthy young and old adults and patients with lung disease. Gottfried and colleagues[134] reported that exponents for the perceived magnitude of resistive loads added to inspiration were significantly reduced in patients with COPD compared to healthy, young adults. Such differences, however, were not observed between patients with asthma and controls.[134,147] In a subsequent series of experiments, Tack and colleagues observed that exponents for both resistive and elastic loads were significantly reduced in older adults (> 60 years) compared to younger adults (< 31 years).[148,149] These latter findings are consistent with the general decline in sensory and perceptual functions observed with increasing age,[150] and conclusions were made that the "blunted" perceptual performance in both older individuals and patients with COPD may be due to impairment in

Table 7. Representative Exponents for Power Functions
Relating Subjective Magnitude to Stimulus Magnitude

Continuum	Measured exponent	Stimulus condition
Brightness	0.50	Very brief flash
Smell	0.60	Heptane
Loudness	0.67	3,150 Hz signal
Respiration	0.80	Resistive loads (young adults)
Respiration	0.95	Elastic loads (young adults)
Vibration	0.95	60 Hz on finger
Visual line length	1.00	Projected line
Respiration	1.05	Breath-hold discomfort
Respiration	1.20	Inspired lung volume
Taste	1.30	Sucrose
Temperature	1.50	Warmth on arm
Respiration	1.54	Ventilation (normal)
Saturation	1.70	Red
Force of handgrip	1.70	Hand dynamometer
Respiration	1.70	Static respiratory forces
Electric shock	3.50	Current through fingers

Adapted from Baird JC, Noma E. Fundamentals of Scaling and Psychophysics. New York, J Wiley & Sons, 1978, with permission.

the central nervous system processing of respiratory-related signals.[134,143,144,151]

Gottfried and colleagues[144] replicated their initial findings in patients with COPD and similar-aged controls, but the possibility of a confound of chronological age on psychophysical scaling results in patients with lung disease was pursued further in three additional studies. Ward and Stubbing[52] found that exponents for the perceived magnitude of both resistive and elastic loads computed in young adults were greater compared to those for patients, but no difference was observed between exponents for patients and age-matched controls. In more recent experiments, Mahler and colleagues[145,152] found similarities in the average size of exponents for resistive loads in patients with airflow obstruction, and for elastic loads in patients with interstitial lung disease, and healthy, age-matched controls (Figures 7 and 8). Further research is needed to resolve the differential manner in which chronological age and underlying pathophysiology yield similar psychophysical outcomes.

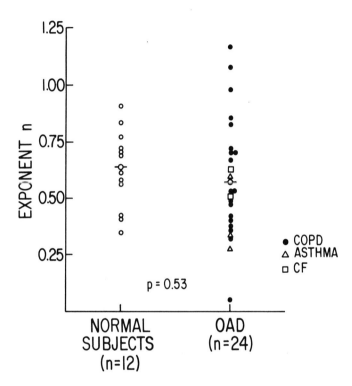

Figure 7: *Individual and mean (-○-) exponents for added resistances in normal subects and patients with obstructive airway disease. (From Mahler DA, Rosiello RA, Harver A, et al. Comparison of clinical dyspnea ratings and psychophysical measurements of respiratory sensation in obstructive airway disease. Am Rev Respir Dis 1987; 135: 1229-1233, with permission.)*

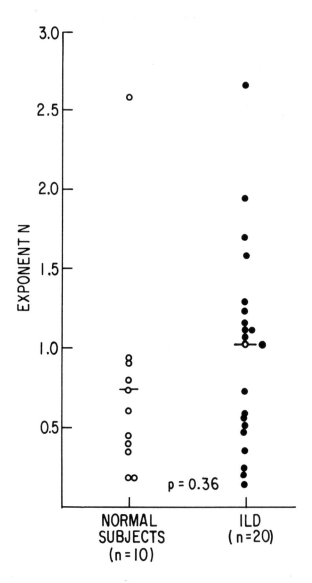

Figure 8: *Individual and mean (-○-) exponents for mouth pressure for elastic loads added to breathing in normal subjects and patients with interstitial lung disease. (From Mahler DA, Harver A, Rosiello R, et al. Measurement of respiratory sensation in interstitial lung disease: evaluation of clinical dyspnea ratings and magnitude scaling. Chest 1989; 96:767-771, with permission.)*

C. Multidimensional Scaling Approaches

Despite considerable literature on the psychophysics of respiratory sensations, the psychophysical relations between stimulus and sensation in breathing remain largely unspecified.[153,154] For example, agreement on the sensory attributes that underlie psychophysical decisions has not emerged. It is difficult to see how direct scaling approaches might provide evidence favoring certain attributes of sensory experience over any other. Magnitude scaling requires that the subject attend to a single sensory aspect of breathing closely specified by the experimenter's instructions. In direct scaling, therefore, the observer may be forced to collapse a number of different dimensions of sensory experience onto a single strength-of-sensation dimension.[155,156]

An alternative set of methods designed to help uncover the possible parameters or dimensions of sensory experience are those relying on clustering and multidimensional scaling algorithms.[157,158] Such techniques recently have proven valuable in the study of pain,[155,156] and have been used to help uncover the organization of sensory experiences surrounding respiratory sensations elicited by various breathing maneuvers.[153,154] With these methods, the observer represents his or her perceptual world not by judgments of perceived magnitude, but by rating the relative similarity between pairs of stimulus objects,[153] or by choosing descriptors of sensory experience from among a list that applies to specific stimulus objects.[154] Subsequent analyses provide either clusters (nests) or "maps" of variables in terms of the degree of perceived similarity among the stimuli or descriptors.

Harver and colleagues[153] examined the perceived similarity among respiratory sensations elicited by nine breathing maneuvers, including inspiring and expiring against a closed airway, inspiring and expiring against two levels of resistive loads, and inspiring against two levels of elastic loads. Analyses were conducted among ratings of similarity made between all possible pairs of stimuli. The results of both cluster and mutidimensional scaling analyses were complementary, and provided evidence that individuals organize sensations elicited by these maneuvers primarily along a single sensory continuum or dimension, namely, the degree or magnitude of impedance opposing respiration (Figure 9). The relative location of breathing maneuvers within the "space" provides an empirical context in which to consider the integration or gating of signals related to pressure or tension, flow, displacement, and effort.

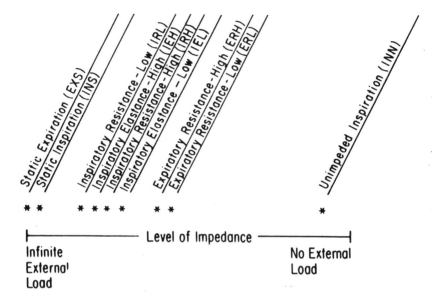

Figure 9: *Multidimensional scaling outcome of relative perceived similarity judgments obtained for pairs of breathing sensations. Each point in the space ("map") is associated with a fixed, scaled location along the horixontal axis. (From Harver A, Baird JC, McGovern JF, et al. Grouping and multidimensional organization of respiratory sensations. Percept Psychophys 1988; 44:285-292, with permission.)*

More recently, Simon et al.[154] examined the similarities of sensory experience elicited by eight breathing maneuvers, including breathholding, breathing against resistive and elastic loads, and exercise in 30 healthy subjects. After each maneuver, subjects chose from among a list of 19 phrases those that described the sensations experienced during the maneuver. Nine clusters of descriptors emerged from the analysis. Some clusters were associated with different stimuli; rapid and heavy breathing were associated with exercise; and rapid and effortful breathing were associated with carbon dioxide stimulation. Breathholding was associated with air hunger. Based on the different groupings of descriptors that emerged for the different stimuli examined, descriptions of breathlessness may reflect different qualities of sensation and not simply variations in the intensity or quantity of sensation.[154] Subsequent research will be needed to confirm such an hypothesis.

VI. Load Perception and Dyspnea

The previous review of respiratory psychophysics indicates clearly that detection thresholds and mathematical relationships between stimulus-sensation pairs can be readily determined for extrapulmonary resistive and elastic loads in healthy young and old adults, as well as in patients with lung disease. Many of these investigations have provided original evidence for various neurophysiological mechanisms that could underlie load perception. On the other hand, the relationship between psychophysical outcomes and the symptom of dyspnea remains controversial.[14,20,23,30] The extent to which extrapulmonary resistive and elastic loads either duplicate (in normal subjects) or replicate (in patients with lung disease) internal flow and volume limitations germane to the sensory experience of difficult, labored breathing is quite speculative.

A. Psychophysical Outcomes and Dyspnea

An issue of theoretical importance that has attracted little empirical testing is the actual relationship between psychophysical outcomes and the symptom of dyspnea in patients with lung disease. In an early experiment conducted along these lines, Wood and colleagues[159] described a lack of correlation between symptoms and sensory acuity on a resistive load detection task in patients with chronic lung disease. Results from more recent investigations provide evidence for the independence between the perceived magnitude of sensations elicited by mechanical loads and sensations associated with internal loads (dyspnea). For example, correlations among clinical dyspnea ratings, lung function, and exponents for resistive loads were compared in 24 patients with obstructive airway disease.[145] Significant correlation coefficients (r) were obtained among the clinical methods (range of r values, 0.71–0.83), and dyspnea scores were significantly correlated with lung function (range of r values, 0.43–0.49). However, dyspnea scores and exponents for resistive loads were not significantly correlated (range of r values, 0.07–0.25), and correlations between lung function and exponents were small and non-significant (range of r values, 0.01–0.11). In other words, the perceived magnitude of acute increases in airway resistance were not related to clinical scores of dyspnea. Results of more complicated analytic procedures (factor analysis) provide additional support for the conclusion that clinical ratings of dyspnea and the perceived magnitude of resistive loads are not equivalent and therefore should not be interchanged.[160] In a subsequent investigation, interrelationships among clinical rating scales, psychophysical outcomes for elastic loads, and physiological function demonstrated that these assessment approaches provide distinct information in patients with symptomatic interstitial lung disease.[152]

Together, results of investigations directly comparing different approaches to the assessment of respiratory sensation in patients with lung disease suggest that psychophysical sensitivity is not synonymous with the sensory experience of dyspnea. This conclusion is consistent with the distinction made by Pennebaker and Hoover[64] between "detection" (broadly conceived) and "perception." In their analysis, psychophysical outcomes are highly dependent on sensory information arising from stimulation of physiological receptors.[41] In the psychophysical context, therefore, judgments of internal states are directly proportional to such stimulation because all other sources of information are assumed to be held constant.[41,64] Perception, on the other hand, is based on the active processing of multiple sources of information, and judgments of sensation are shaded by past experiences and by large numbers of competing internal and external sensory signals.[37,64] The distinction between detection and perception could account for the lack of relationship observed between psychophysical outcomes and (clinical ratings of) dyspnea.

B. Extrapulmonary Loads and Lung Disease

In an editorial to the proceedings of an international symposium on mechanical loads and breathing published in 1974,[161] the editors noted that "common to many conditions causing breathlessness is a disturbance of the mechanics of breathing," and further that "an understanding of the way in which the act of breathing is affected by added mechanical loads is essential to an appreciation of these common clinical problems." Subsequently, numerous papers have reviewed loaded breathing experiments conducted in healthy subjects and patients with chronic lung disease, and summarized the considerable scientific advances made in the areas of respiratory mechanics and the control of breathing.[162,163] In many of these reviews, the limits of extrapulmonary loads as an analog for examining the functional changes of the respiratory apparatus consequent to disease are addressed. These limits are strikingly relevant also for discussions of the comparability of the sensory experiences in lung disease and load perception.

Internal loads frequently are associated with complex and localized stressors not produced by mechanical loads.[164] Unlike external loads, pulmonary disease seldom effects the lungs uniformly but results in an invariant set of mechanical aberrations.[162] Such invariance may result in unique sources of sensory information used in processing respiratory sensations that are not represented in experimental situations. Mechanical loads may not fully duplicate the pattern of mechanoreceptor stimulation produced by lung disease, and temporal factors may serve to further reduce the similarity between the acute physiological and behavioral responses to extrapulmonary loads in the laboratory and those of the patient with lung disease.[162] Finally, no standards exist for directly comparing the differential quantities of resistance and elastance on either reflexive or behavioral responses.[165]

VII. Summary and Conclusions

This chapter has reviewed the phenomenon of dyspnea, both as a symptom and as a sensory experience, focusing on clinical, physiological, and behavioral aspects of the dyspneic patient. It has shown that the lack of a precise definition of the symtom of dyspnea, the large and variable nature of the conditions in which dyspnea is a complaint, and the discrete respiratory sensations used, in part, to model the symptom of dyspnea, contribute to the obscure nature of a relatively common problem where little agreement is evident. It presented a number of demographic, sociocultural, and individual difference variables that affect symptom reporting, and emphasized the multidimensional character of the symptom of dyspnea. It reviewed in some detail both indirect and direct psychophysical approaches to assess sensory experience, and reviewed results from the application of these procedures, as well as of alternative procedures (signal detection and multidimensional approaches), to extrapulmonary load perception. Finally, the relationship between load perception and dyspnea was addressed, and distinction was made between the detection and perception of internal states to account for the apparent lack of agreement between psychophysical outcomes and the sensory experience of dyspnea.

Dyspnea is a synthetic sensation, like thirst or hunger, that results from active processing of primary respiratory signals (e.g., metabolic demand, ventilation achieved), as well as multiple collateral physiological signals (e.g., fatigue, muscular aching) and psychological states (e.g., memory, affect). If breathing is "a strange phenomenon of life, caught midway between the conscious and unconscious,"[166] then research on the symptom of dyspnea, perhaps somewhat paradoxically, may yield meaningful hypotheses about the relationships between the act of breathing and the control of breathing.

It is likely, in this context, that sensory psychophysics will continue to provide original insight to the interactions between behavioral responses and ventilatory control. For example, variations in the severity of dyspnea in patients with comparable degress of airway obstruction could be examined in terms of the differences (variability) in perceptual responses on psychophysical scaling tasks.[22,30,167] Other techniques such as magnitude-matching, signal detection, and multidimensional scaling could be called upon to explore more directly the non-sensory and long-term effects of chronic pulmonary disease on the perception of sensory experience.

At the same time, there is a need to continue to recognize the limits of investigations designed to assess the intensity or similarities of subjective sensations elicited by standardized, laboratory stimuli. In the literature on pain, for example, sensory psychophysics has overshadowed the role of the motivational and affective components of the pain experience.[168] But regardless of the approach adopted to investigate an increasingly common and severely disabling clinical problem, it may be wise to heed the advice of MacKenzie,[169] who nearly 100 years ago cautioned that "when making an observation upon any symptom, care should be taken to record nothing beyond what, strictly speaking, the facts warrant."

References

1. U.S. Public Health Service. Epidemiology of respiratory diseases. Task force report on state of knowledge, problems, and needs. Washington, D.C.: U.S. Government Printing Office, 1981. DHEW Publication No. (NIH)81-2019.

2. U.S. Public Health Service. Tenth report of the director. National Heart, Lung and Blood Institute ten-year review and five-year plan. Volume 3. Lung diseases. Washington, D.C.: U.S. Government Printing Office, 1984. DHEW Publication No. (NIH)84-2358.

3. Bennett ED, Jayson MIV, Rubenstein D, et al. The ability of man to detect non-elastic loads to breathing. Clin Sci 1962; 23:155-162.

4. Campbell EJM, Freedman S, Smith PS, et al. The ability of man to detect added elastic loads to breathing. Clin Sci 1961; 20:223-231.

5. Campbell EJM, Howell JBL. The sensation of breathlessness. Br Med Bull 1963; 19:36-40.

6. Guz A. Respiratory sensations in man. Br Med Bull 1977; 33:175-177.

7. Killian KJ. The objective measurement of breathlessness. Chest 1985; 88(suppl):84S-90S.

8. Bakers JHCM, Tenney SM. The perception of some sensations associated with breathing. Respir Physiol 1970; 10:85-92.

9. Altose MD, Cherniack N, Fishman AP. Respiratory sensations and dyspnea. J Appl Physiol 1985; 58:1051-1054.

10. Burki NK. Dyspnea. Clin Chest Med 1980; 1:47-55.

11. Burki NK. Dyspnea. Lung 1987; 165:269-277.

12. Campbell EJM, Guz A. Breathlessness. In: Hornbein TF (ed). Regulation of Breathing, Part 2. New York, Marcel Dekker, 1981; 1181-1195.

13. Carrieri VK, Janson-Bjerklie S, Jacobs S. The sensation of dyspnea: a review. Heart Lung 1984; 13:436-447.

14. Cockroft A, Adams L. Measurement and mechanisms of breathlessness. Bull Eur Physiopathol Respir 1986; 22:85-92.

15. Gold WM. Dyspnea. In: Blacklow RS (ed). MacBryde's Signs and Symptoms, 6th Edition. Philadelphia, JB Lippincott, 1983; 335-348.

16. Janson-Bjerklie S, Carrieri VK, Hudes M. The sensations of pulmonary dyspnea. Nurs Res 1986; 35:154-159.

17. Jones NL. Dyspnea in exercise. Med Sci Sports Exerc 1984; 16:14-19.

18. Killian KJ, Campbell EJM. Dyspnea. In: Roussos C, Macklem PT (eds). The Thorax, Part B. New York, Marcel Dekker, 1985; 787-828.

19. Mahler DA. Dyspnea: Diagnosis and management. Clin Chest Med 1987; 8:215-230.

20. Wasserman K, Casaburi R. Dyspnea: physiological and pathophysiological mechanisms. Ann Rev Med 1988; 39:503-515.

21. Killian KJ, Jones NL. The use of exercise testing and other methods in the investigation of dyspnea. Clin Chest Med 1984; 5:99-108.

22. Altose MD. Psychophysics—an approach to the study of respiratory sensation and the assessment of dyspnea. Am Rev Respir Dis 1987; 135:1227-1228.

23. The enigma of breathlessness (editorial). Lancet 1986; i:891-892.

24. Killian KJ. Assessment of dyspnoea. Eur Respir J 1988; 1:195-197.

25. Altose MD. Assessment and management of breathlessness. Chest 1985; 88(suppl):77S-83S.

26. Zechman FW Jr, Wiley RL. Afferent inputs to breathing: respiratory sensation. In: Cherniack NS, Widdicombe JG (eds). Handbook of Phys-

iology, Section 3: The Respiratory System. Bethesda, American Physiological Society, 1986; 449-474.

27. Comroe JH Jr. Summing up. In: Howell JBL, Campbell EJM (eds). Breathlessness. Oxford, Blackwell Scientific Publications, 1966; 233-238.

28. Wasserman K. The chairman's postconference reflections. Am Rev Respir Dis 1984; 129(suppl):S1-S2.

29. Sivraprasad R, Payne CB Jr. Nonpulmonary causes of dyspnea. Radiol Clin North Am 1984; 22:463-465.

30. Killian KJ, Campbell EJM. Dyspnea and excercise. Annu Rev Physiol 1983; 45:465-479.

31. Cervero F, Morrison JFB (eds). Progress in Brain Research (Vol 67): Visceral Sensation. Amsterdam, Elsevier, 1986.

32. Reed SD, Harver A, Katkin ES. Interoception. In: Cacioppo JT, Tassinary LG (eds). Principles of Psychophysiology: Physical, Social, and Inferential Elements. Cambridge, Cambridge University Press, in press.

33. Geldard FA. The Human Senses, 2nd Edition. New York, J Wiley & Sons, 1972.

34. Boring EG. Sensation and Perception in the History of Experimental Psychology. New York, Appleton-Century-Crofts Inc., 1942.

35. Pennebaker JW, Gonsler-Frederick L, Cox DJ, et al. The perception of general vs. specific visceral activity and the regulation of health-related behavior. In: Katkin ES, Manuck SB (eds). Advances in Behavioral Medicine (Vol 1): Greenwich, CT, JAI Press, 1985; 165-198.

36. James W. What is an emotion? Mind 1884; 9:188-205.

37. Pennebaker JW. The Psychology of Physical Symptoms. New York, Springer-Verlag, 1982.

38. Pennebaker JW, Epstein D. Implicit psychophysiology: effects of common beliefs and idiosyncratic physiological responses on symptom reporting. J Pers 1983; 51:468-496.

39. Mechanic D. The epidemiology of illness behavior and its relationship to physical and psychological distress. In: Mechanic D (ed). Symptoms, Illness Behavior, and Help-Seeking. New York, Neale Watson Academic Publications, Inc., 1982; 1-24.

40. Leventhal H, Nerenz DR, Straus A. Self-regulation and the mechanisms for symptom appraisal. In: Mechanic D (ed). Symptoms, Illness Behavior, and Help-Seeking. New York, Neale Watson Academic Publications, Inc., 1982; 55-86.

41. Pennebaker JW, Brittingham GL. Environmental and sensory cues affecting the perception of physical symptoms. In: Baum A, Singer JE (eds). Advances in Environmental Psychology. Hillsdale, NJ, Laurence Erlbaum Associates, 1982; 115-136.

42. Whitehead WE, Busch CM, Heller BR, et al. Social learning influences on menstrual symptoms and illness behavior. Health Psychol 1986; 5: 13-23.

43. Turk DC, Rudy TE. Toward an empirically derived taxonomy of chronic pain patients: integration of psychological assessment data. J Consult Clin Psychol 1988; 56:233-238.

44. Dudley DL, Sitzman J, Rugg M. Psychiatric aspects of patients with chronic obstructive pulmonary disease. In: Thompson WL, Thompson TL II (eds). Advances in Psychosomatic Medicine (Vol 14). Basel, Switzerland, S Karger, 1985; 64-77.
45. Stedman's Medical Dictionary, 24th Edition. Baltimore, Williams & Wilkins, 1982.
46. Blacklow RS. The study of symptoms. In: Blacklow RS (ed). MacBryde's Signs and Symptoms, 6th Edition. Philadelphia, JB Lippincott, 1983; 1-16.
47. Howell JBL, Campbell EJM (eds). Breathlessness. Oxford, Blackwell Scientific Publications, 1966.
48. Oliven A, Kelsen SG, Deal EC Jr, et al. Respiratory pressure sensation. Am Rev Respir Dis 1985; 132:1214-1218.
49. Poon C. Effects of inspiratory resistive load on respiratory control in hypercapnia and exercise. J Appl Physiol 1989; 66:2391-2399.
50. Poon C. Effects of inspiratory elastic load on respiratory control in hypercapnia and exercise. J Appl Physiol 1989; 66:2400-2406.
51. Cherniack NS, Chonan T, Altose MD. Respiratory sensations and the voluntary control of breathing. In: von Euler C, Katz-Salamon M (eds). Respiratory Psychophysiology. New York, Stockton Press, 1988; 35-45.
52. Ward ME, Stubbing DG. Effect of chronic lung disease on the perception of added inspiratory loads. Am Rev Respir Dis 1985; 132:652-656.
53. Heim E, Blaser A, Waidelich E. Dyspnea: psychophysiologic relationships. Psychosom Med 1972; 34:405-423.
54. Welch MH. Obstructive diseases. In: Guenter CA, Welch MH (eds). Pulmonary Medicine, 2nd Edition. Philadelphia, JB Lippincott, 1982; 663-793.
55. Burns BH. Breathlessness in depression. Br J Psychiatry 1971; 119:39-45.
56. Comroe JH Jr. Dyspnea. Mod Concepts Cardiovasc Dis 1956; 25:347-349.
57. Kinsman RA, Fernandez E, Schocket M, et al. Multidimensional analysis of the symptoms of chronic bronchitis and emphysema. J Behav Med 1983; 6:339-357.
58. Kinsman RA, Luparello T, O'Banion K, et al. Multidimensional analysis of the subjective symptomatology of asthma. Psychosom Med 1973; 35:250-267.
59. Kinsman RA, O'Banion K, Resnikoff P, et al. Subjective symptoms of acute asthma within a heterogeneous sample of asthmatics. J Allergy Clin Immunol 1973; 52:284-296.
60. Kinsman RA, Yaroush RA, Fernandez E, et al. Symptoms and experience in chronic bronchitis and emphysema. Chest 1983; 83:755-761.
61. Creer TL. Asthma Therapy. New York, Springer, 1979.
62. Creer TL, Renne CM, Chai H. The application of behavioral techniques to childhood asthma. In: Russo DC, Varni JW (eds). Behavioral Pediatrics: Research and Practice. New York, Plenum Press, 1982:27-66.
63. Creer TL. Response: self-management psychology and the treatment of childhood asthma. J Allergy Clin Immunol 1983; 72:607-610.

64. Pennebaker JW, Hoover CW. Visceral perception versus visceral detection: disentangling methods and assumptions. Biofeedback Self Regul 1984; 9:339-352.
65. Glauser FL (ed). Signs and symptoms in pulmonary medicine. Philadelphia, JB Lippincott, 1983.
66. Mahler DA, Barlow PB, Matthay RA. Chronic obstructive pulmonary disease. Clin Geriatr Med 1986; 2:285-312.
67. Des Jardins TR. Clinical Manifestations of Respiratory Disease. Chicago, Year Book Medical Publishers, Inc., 1984.
68. Gift AG, Plaut SM, Jacox A. Psychologic and physiologic factors related to dyspnea in subjects with chronic obstructive pulmonary disease. Heart Lung 1986; 15:595-601.
69. Chai H, Purcell K, Brady K, et al. Therapeutic and investigational evaluation of asthmatic children. J Allergy 1968; 41:23-36.
70. Kotses H, Harver A, Creer TL, et al. Measures of asthma severity recorded by patients. J Asthma 1988; 25:373-376.
71. Rubinfeld AF, Pain MCF. Perception of asthma. Lancet 1976; i:882-884.
72. Burdon JGW, Juniper EF, Killian KJ, et al. The perception of breathlessness in asthma. Am Rev Respir Dis 1982; 126:825-828.
73. Couriel JM, Demis T, Olinsky A. The perception of asthma. Aust Paediatr J 1986; 22:45-47.
74. Orehek J, Beaupre A, Badier M, et al. Perception of airway tone by asthmatic individuals. Bull Eur Physiopathol Respir 1982; 18:601-606.
75. Parker SR. Future directions in behavioral research related to lung diseases. Ann Behav Med 1985; 7:21-25.
76. Parker SR. Behavioral science aspects of COPD: current status and future directions. In: McSweeny AJ, Grant I (eds). Chronic Obstructive Pulmonary Disease: A Behavioral Perspective. New York, Marcel Dekker, 1988; 279-303.
77. Speilberger CD, Gorsuch RL, Lushene RE. Manual for the State- Trait Anxiety Inventory. Palo Alto, CA, Consulting Psychologist Press, 1970.
78. Beck AT, Rush AJ, Shaw BF. Cognitive Therapy of Depression. New York, Guilford Publications, Inc., 1979.
79. Bergner M, Bobbit RA, Pollard WE. The sickness impact profile: validation of a health status measure. Med Care 1976; 14:57-67.
80. Derogatis LR. SCL-90 Administration, Scoring, and Procedures Manuals for the Revised Version. Baltimore, Leonard R. Derogatis, 1977.
81. McNair DM, Lorr M, Droppleman LF. EDITS Manual for the Profile of Mood States. San Diego, Educational and Industrial Testing Service, 1971.
82. Fanshel F, Bush JW. A Health Status Index and its applications to health services outcomes. Oper Res 1970; 18:1021-1066.
83. Jones PW, Baveystock CM, Littlejohns P. Relationships between general health measured with the Sickness Impact Profile and respiratory symptoms, physiological measures, and mood in patients with chronic airflow limitation. Am Rev Respir Dis 1989; 140:1538-1543.

84. Keller C. Predicting the performance of daily activities of patients with chronic lung disease. Percept Mot Skills 1986; 63:647-651.
85. Orenstein DM, Nixon PA, Ross EA, et al. The Quality of Well-Being in cystic fibrosis. Chest 1989; 95:344-347.
86. Prigatano GP, Wright EC, Levin D. Quality of life and its predictors in patients with mild hypoxemia and chronic obstructive pulmonary disease. Arch Intern Med 1984; 144:1613-1619.
87. Rosser R, Guz A. Psychological approaches to breathlessness and its treatment. J Psychosom Res 1981; 25:439-447.
88. Dudley DL, Martin CJ, Holmes TH. Dyspnea: psychologic and physiologic observations. J Psychosom Res 1968; 11:325-339.
89. Bass C, Gardner W. Emotional influences on breathing and breathlessness. J Psychosom Res 1985; 29:599-609.
90. Dales RE, Spitzer WO, Schechter MT, et al. The influence of psychological status on respiratory symptom reporting. Am Rev Respir Dis 1989; 139:1459-1463.
91. Dahlstrom WG, Welsh GS, Dahlstrom LE. An MMPI Handbook, Revised Edition. Minneapolis, University of Minnesota, 1972.
92. Agle DP, Baum GL. Psychological aspects of chronic obstructive pulmonary disease. Med Clin N Am 1977; 61:749-758.
93. Greenberg GD, Ryan JJ, Bourlier PF. Psychological and neuropsychological aspects of COPD. Psychosomatics 1985; 26:29-33.
94. Oswald NC, Waller RE, Drinkwater J. Relationship between breathlessness and anxiety in asthma and bronchitis: a comparative study. Br Med J 1970; 2:14-17.
95. Prigatano GP, Grant I. Neuropsychological correlates of COPD. In: McSweeny AJ, Grant I (eds). Chronic Obstructive Pulmonary Disease: A Behavioral Perspective. New York, Marcel Dekker, 1988; 39-57.
96. Reitan RM, Davison LA. Clinical Neuropsychology: Current Status and Applications. Washington, DC, VH Winston and Sons, 1974.
97. Reitan RM. Theoretical and methodological bases of the Halstead-Reitan Neuropsychological Test Battery. In: Grant I, Adams KM (eds). Neuropsychological Assessment of Neuropsychiatric Disorders. New York, Oxford University Press, 1986; 3-30.
98. Stevens SS. Perceptual magnitude and its measurement. In: Carterette EC, Friedman MP (eds). Handbook of Perception (Vol 2). New York, Academic Press, 1974; 361-389.
99. Carterette EC, Friedman MP (eds). Handbook of Perception (Vol 2). New York, Academic Press, 1974.
100. Baird JC, Noma E. Fundamentals of Scaling and Psychophysics. New York, J Wiley & Sons, 1978.
101. Coren S, Porac C, Ward LM. Sensation and Perception, 2nd Edition. Orlando, FL, Academic Press, Inc., 1984.
102. D'Amato MR. Experimental Psychology: Methodology, Psychophysics, and Learning. New York, McGraw-Hill Book Co., 1970.
103. Gescheider GA. Psychophysics: Method and Theory. Hillsdale, NJ, Lawrence Erlbuam Associates, 1976.

104. Stevens SS. Psychophysics: Introduction to its Perceptual, Neural, and Social Prospects. New York, J Wiley & Sons, 1975.
105. Boring EG. A History of Experimental Psychology, 2nd Edition. New York, Appleton-Century-Crofts, 1950.
106. Rosner BS, Goff WR. Electrical responses of the nervous system and subjective scales of intensity. In: Neff WD (ed). Contributions to Sensory Physiology (Vol 2). New York, Academic Press, 1967; 169-221.
107. Stevens SS. The direct estimation of sensory magnitudes— loudness. Am J Psychol 1956; 69:1-25.
108. Guilford JP. Psychometric Methods, 2nd Edition. New York, McGraw-Hill Book Co., 1954.
109. Katz-Salamon M. Respiratory psychophysics: a methodological overview. In: von Euler C, Katz-Salamon M (eds). Respiratory Psychophysics. New York, Stockton Press, 1988; 65-78.
110. Swets JA. The relative operating characteristic in psychology. Science 1973; 182:990-1000.
111. Borg GAV. A category scale with ratio properties for intermodal and interindividual comparisons. In: Geissler H, Petzold P (eds). Psychophysical Judgment and the Process of Perception. Amsterdam, North-Holland, 1982; 25-34.
112. Borg GAV. Psychophysical bases of perceived exertion. Med Sci Sports Exerc 1982; 14:377-381.
113. Stevens SS. Matching functions between loudness and ten other continua. Percept Psychophys 1966; 1:5-8.
114. Stevens JC. Magnitude matching: a new method to assess sensory magnitude. In: Geissler H, Petzold P (eds). Psychophysical Judgment and the Process of Perception. Amsterdam, North-Holland, 1982; 17-24.
115. Gescheider GA. Psychophysical scaling. Annu Rev Psychol 1988; 39: 169-200.
116. Baird JC. A cognitive theory of psychophysics. II. Fechner's law and Stevens' law. Scand J Psychol 1970; 11:89-102.
117. Teghtsoonian R. On the exponents in Stevens' law and the constant in Ekman's law. Psychol Rev 1971; 78:71-80.
118. Stevens SS. The psychophysics of sensory function. Am Sci 1960; 48: 226-253.
119. Stevens SS. Neural events and the psychophysical law. Science 1970; 170:1043-1050.
120. Borg G, Diamant H, Strom L, et al. The relation between neural and perceptual intensity: a comparative study on the neural and psychophysical response to taste stimuli. J Physiol 1967; 192:13-20.
121. Borg G. Simple rating methods for estimation of perceived exertion. In: Borg G (ed). Physical Work and Effort. Oxford, Pergamon Press, 1977; 39-47.
122. Borg GAV. Perceived exertion: a note on "history" and methods. Med Sci Sports 1973; 5:90-93.
123. Marks LE, Borg G, Ljunggren G. Individual differences in perceived

exertion assessed by two new methods. Percept Psychophys 1983; 34: 280-288.
124. Harver A, Tenney SM, Baird JC. A cautionary note on the interpretation of the power law for respiratory effort. Am Rev Respir Dis 1986; 133: 341-342.
125. Gottfried SB, Altose MD, Kelsen SG, et al. The perception of changes in airflow resistance in normal subjects and patients with chronic airways obstruction. Chest 1978; 73(suppl):286-288.
126. Altose MD, Dimarco AF, Gottfried SB, et al. The sensation of respiratory muscle force. Am Rev Respir Dis 1982; 126:807-811.
127. Killian KJ, Mahutte CK, Campbell EJM. Magnitude scaling of externally added loads to breathing. Am Rev Respir Dis 1981; 123:12-15.
128. Killian KJ, Bucens DD, Campbell EJM. Effect of breathing patterns on the perceived magnitude of added loads to breathing. J Appl Physiol 1982; 52:578-584.
129. Muza SR, McDonald S, Zechman FW. Comparison of subjects' perception of inspiratory and expiratory resistance. J Appl Physiol 1984; 56: 211-216.
130. Burki NK. Detection of added respiratory loads in patients with restrictive lung disease. Am Rev Respir Dis 1985; 132:1210-1213.
131. Burki NK, Mitchell K, Chaudhary BA, et al. The ability of asthmatics to detect added resistive loads. Am Rev Respir Dis 1978; 117:71-75.
132. Stubbing DG, Killian KJ, Campbell EJM. Weber's law and resistive load detection. Am Rev Respir Dis 1983; 127:5-7.
133. Wiley RL, Zechman FW. Perception of added airflow resistance in humans. Respir Physiol 1966; 2:73-87.
134. Gottfried SB, Altose MD, Kelsen SG, et al. Perception of changes in airflow resistance in obstructive pulmonary disorders. Am Rev Respir Dis 1981; 124:566-570.
135. Chaudhary BA, Burki NK. The effects of airway anesthesia on detection of added inspiratory elastic loads. Am Rev Respir Dis 1980; 122: 635-639.
136. Hudgel DW, Cooperson DM, Kinsman RA. Recognition of added resistive loads in asthma. Am Rev Respir Dis 1982; 126:121-125.
137. Tiller J, Pain M, Biddle N. Anxiety disorder and the perception of inspiratory resistive loads. Chest 1987; 91:547-551.
138. Narbed PG, Marcer D, Howell JBL. The contribution of the accelerating phase of inspiratory flow to resistive load detection in man. Clin Sci 1982; 62:367-372.
139. Narbed PG, Marcer D, Howell JBL, et al. A signal detection theory analysis of the effects of chest cage restriction upon the detection of inspiratory resistive loads. Clin Sci 1983; 64:417-421.
140. Bonnel AM, Mathiot MJ, Grimaud C. Inspiratory and expiratory resistive load detection in normal and asthmatic subjects. Respiration 1985; 48:12-23.
141. Harver A, Kotses H. Perception of static respiratory forces in young and old subjects. Percept Psychophys 1987; 41:449-454.

142. Oliven A, Kelsen SG, Deal EC Jr, et al. Effect of respiratory sensation on load compensation and CO_2 retention in patients with chronic airflow obstruction. Trans Assoc Am Physicians 1982; 95:319-324.
143. Tack M, Altose MD, Cherniack NS. Effects of aging on sensation of respiratory force and displacement. J Appl Physiol 1983; 55:1433-1440.
144. Gottfried SB, Redline S, Altose MD. Respiratory sensation in chronic obstructive pulmonary disease. Am Rev Respir Dis 1985; 132:954-959.
145. Mahler DA, Rosiello RA, Harver A, et al. Comparison of clinical dyspnea ratings and psychophysical measurements of respiratory sensation in obstructive airway disease. Am Rev Respir Dis 1987; 135:1229-1233.
146. Harver A. Constancy of individual exponents for category production of inspired lung volume. Percept Mot Skills 1987; 65:779-785.
147. Burki N. Effects of bronchodilation on magnitude estimation of added resistive loads in asthmatic subjects. Am Rev Respir Dis 1984; 129:225-229.
148. Tack M, Altose MD, Cherniack NS. Effect of aging on respiratory sensations produced by elastic loads. J Appl Physiol 1981; 50:844-850.
149. Tack M, Altose MD, Cherniack NS. Effect of aging on the perception of resistive ventilatory loads. Am Rev Respir Dis 1982; 126:463-467.
150. Corso JF. Sensory processes and age effects in normal adults. J Gerontol 1971; 26:90-105.
151. Altose MD, Leitner J, Cherniack NS. Effects of age and respiratory efforts on the perception of resistive ventilatory loads. J Gerontol 1985; 40:147-153.
152. Mahler DA, Harver A, Rosiello R, et al. Measurement of respiratory sensation in interstitial lung disease: evaluation of clinical dyspnea ratings and magnitude scaling. Chest 1989; 96:767-771.
153. Harver A, Baird JC, McGovern JF, et al. Grouping and multidimensional organization of respiratory sensations. Percept Psychophys 1988; 44:285-292.
154. Simon PM, Schwartzstein RM, Weiss JW, et al. Distinguishable sensations of breathlessness induced in normal volunteers. Am Rev Respir Dis 1989; 140:1021-1027.
155. Clark WC. Application of multidimensional scaling to problems in experimental and clinical pain. In: Brown B (ed). Pain Measurement in Man: Neurophysiological Correlates of Pain. Amsterdam, Elsevier, 1984; 349-369.
156. Clark WC, Carroll JT, Yang JC, et al. Multidimensional scaling reveals two dimensions of thermal pain. J Exp Psychol: Hum Percept Perform 1986; 12:103-107.
157. Johnson SC. Hierarchical clustering schemes. Psychometrika 1967; 32:241-254.
158. McGee VE. The multidimensional analysis of "elastic" distances. Br J Math Stat Psychol 1966; 19:181-196.
159. Wood MM, McCarthy PE, Cotes JE. Perception of airway resistance in relation to breathlessness on exertion in chronic lung disease. Scand J Respir 1971; 77(suppl):98-102.

160. Harver A, Mahler DA, Daubenspeck JA, et al. Multivariate support for three distinct approaches to the assessment of respiratory sensation in patients with obstructive lung disease. In: von Euler C, Katz-Salamon M (eds). Respiratory Psychophysiology. New York, Stockton Press, 1988; 103-112.

161. Pengelly LD, Rebuck AS, Campbell EJM (eds). Loaded Breathing. Edinburgh, Churchill Livingstone, 1974.

162. Cherniack NS, Altose MD. Respiratory responses to ventilatory loading. In: Hornbein TF (ed). Regulation of Breathing, Part 2. New York, Marcel Dekker, 1981; 905-964.

163. Rebuck AS, Slutsky AS. Control of breathing in diseases of the respiratory tract and lung. In: Cherniack NS, Widdicombe JG (eds). Handbook of Physiology, Section 3: The Respiratory System. Bethesda, American Physiological Society, 1986; 771-791.

164. Milic-Emili J, Anthonisen N, Bryan AC, et al. Workshop on assessment of respiratory control in humans: V. The use of loads to study ventilatory control. Am Rev Respir Dis 1977; 115:713.

165. Anthonisen NR. Some steady-state effects of respiratory loads. Chest 1976; 70(suppl):168-169.

166. Richards DW. The nature of cardiac and pulmonary disease. Circulation 1953; 7:15-29.

167. Yamamoto H, Inaba S, Nishimura M, et al. Relationship between the ability to detect added resistance at rest and breathlessness during bronchoconstriction in asthmatics. Respiration 1987; 52:42-48.

168. Melzack R. Concepts of pain measurement. In: Melzack R (ed). Pain Measurement and Assessment. New York, Raven Press, 1983; 1-5.

169. MacKenzie J. Symptoms and Their Interpretation. London, Shaw & Sons, 1909.

Chapter 2

Mechanisms of Dyspnea

K.J. Killian and E.J.M. Campbell

From *Dyspnea*, edited by Donald A. Mahler, M.D., © 1990, Futura Publishing Company, Inc., Mount Kisco, NY.

Whenever a new discovery is reported to the scientific world, they say first, "It is probably not true." Thereafter, when the truth of the new proposition has been demonstrated beyond question they say, "Yes, it is true, but it is not important." Finally, when sufficient time has elapsed to fully evidence its importance, they say, "Yes, surely it is important, but it is no longer new."

Montaigne

I. Introduction

Discomfort in the act of breathing occurs in health and in many forms of disease affecting the lungs, heart, or neuromuscular system. When discomfort is experienced with the act of breathing at a level of activity where it is not expected, dyspnea is said to be present. Clinically, severity is related inversely to the intensity of activity; when experienced climbing stairs, walking, or at rest, increasing severity is inferred. Thus, the circumstances under which it occurs are essential components to its recognition. This discomfort arises under many different circumstances, and as many physiological changes can be demonstrated, there has been a natural curiosity to discover if there is some common mechanism (often called the cause). Breathlessness, shortness of breath, and dyspnea are some of the expressions used to describe this discomfort. The variable use of these terms leads to confusion but adopting a narrow definition is not helpful at this time, firstly because common usage has established that the definitions are practically synonymous; and secondly because we do not yet have sufficient understanding to base our terminology on anything more fundamental. Thus, dyspnea is used throughout this chapter in reference to discomfort experienced and associated with the act of breathing. By contrast, the disorders giving rise to dyspnea are both well known and accepted. This results in the use of terms such as cardiac and respiratory dyspnea, fostering the notion that dyspnea is somehow uniquely related to its etiology. In the last twenty years, there has been progress in defining the anatomy, physiology, and psychophysics of dyspnea and in elucidating the mechanisms of its generation.

II. History

Present understanding began with clinical observation; evolved with advances in the chemical and neural control of breathing, the ability to measure the mechanics of breathing, and sensory physiology; and ended with the application of psychophysics in the interaction of all these elements.

A. Dyspnea and Clinical Observation

In the book entitled *Pathology and Diagnosis of Diseases of the Chest*, published in 1940, C.J.B. William[1] described:

> *Dyspnea, difficult or disordered breathing, is the most important general symptom of diseases of the chest, in as much as it implies more or less interruption to the due performance of some part of the great function of the chest respiration. Dyspnea may be caused by circumstances affecting any one or more of the several elements concerned in the function of respiration: viz the blood in the lungs, the air, the machinery of respiration by which these are brought together, and the nervous system through which the impression which prompts the respiratory act is conveyed from the lung to the medulla, and thence to the muscles which move the machinery.*

Thus, the multiple aspects of the problem were identified from an early stage but exploration was often confined to single processes and was unidimensional.

B. Dyspnea and Chemical Control

In 1868, Pfluger[2] noted that hypoxemia and hypercarbia resulted in dyspnea, but considered oxygen the dominant contributor. Dyspnea was ascribed to the lack of free oxygen in the tissues, particularly in the medulla oblongata. Appreciating that alveolar PCO_2 is closely controlled, Miescher-Rusch[3] noted in 1985 that any rise resulted both in accelerated breathing and in dyspnea. Eight years later, Haldane and Smith[4] found that breathing in a closed chamber resulted in dyspnea when CO_2 levels rose by 3% but not until oxygen dropped to 14%. The concept that hydrogen ion as a common stimulus to respiratory activity and dyspnea was introduced by Winterstein[5] in 1910. In 1923 Meakins,[6] representing the culmination of this period, stated that dyspnea is produced by two causes: want of oxygen and carbon dioxide retention.

C. Dyspnea and Neural Reflexes

By 1931 Cullen, Harrison, Calhoun, Wilkins, and Tims[7] were unhappy with the explanation that chemical changes in the blood were the cause of breathlessness and argued that hydrogen ion, oxygen, and carbon dioxide remain largely unchanged in blood during and following exercise, making these factors less tenable as the mechanisms giving rise to dyspnea. One year later, Harrison et al.[8] went on to show that breathing is stimulated by vagally mediated reflexes, reflexes arising in the central vessels (induced by increased pressure), and muscular movements. The role of reflexes in explaining dyspnea was raised by Harrison[9] and by Gesell and Moyer[10] in the same year, 1935. Christie[11] summarized the understanding of this period in an article published in 1938:

> *Though the conditions under which dyspnea occurs are various and manifold, giving rise to an impression of complexity, the fundamental causes are few and relatively simple. They consist of chemical and reflex disturbances. Chemical disturbance would seem to be of minor importance. Dyspnea is usually reflex in origin.*

D. Dyspnea and Mechanics

Ventilation expressed relative to ventilatory capacity and its relationship to dyspnea was recognized by Means[12] in 1924 and popularized by Cournand and Richards in the 1930s.[13,14] The mechanical characteristics of the respiratory system were outlined by Rohrer[15] in the 1920s. About two decades later, Rahn and his colleagues[16] made it possible to measure the forces and impedances involved in the act of breathing in living subjects. The mechanical work of breathing in patients with heart failure was found to be twice as much at rest and 3 to 4 times as much during exercise as that found in normal subjects.[17] Cherniack and Snidal[18] showed that the work of breathing in patients with emphysema was similarly increased. In 1954 Marshall, Stone, and Christie[19] suggested that dyspnea was related to transpulmonary pressure and not to the work of breathing. Although consensus as to the particular mechanical factor giving rise to breathlessness did not emerge, the idea that the mechanics of respiration are important to the sensation of dyspnea persists to the present day.

E. Dyspnea and Oxygen Cost of Breathing

Oxygen cost of breathing increases when ventilation is increased and when the impedance to the action of the respiratory muscles is increased.[20–23] In 1958, McIlroy[24] concluded that dyspnea occurred when the respiratory muscles incur an oxygen debt.

F. Dyspnea and Length/Tension Inappropriateness

Campbell and Howell[25] suggested in 1963 that an imbalance in the relationship between tension and displacement in respiratory muscles might be the neurophysiological mechanism giving rise to dyspnea. Tension mediated by tendon organs, and length (volume or flow) mediated by muscle spindles and joint receptors, is transmitted to the central nervous system. The central processing of these signals provides a viable neurophysiological mechanism for the sensation. At that time, gamma efferent motor activity to intrafusal muscle fibers (spindles) was considered as a possible primary motor innervation to muscle. The increase in spindle discharge resulting from the stretching of the nuclear bag would cause afferent fiber stimulation, and would increase alpha motor neurone activity reflexly. Alpha motor activity acted as a follow up to a length servo system. Later, Campbell[26,27] substituted length/length for length/tension. An imbalance between programmed length change and achieved length change would trigger dyspnea, according to this hypothesis.

G. Summary

There is general agreement that hypoxemia, hypercapnia, and increased hydrogen ion concentration cause dyspnea; that increasing ventilation as a consequence of reflex activity arising in the muscles, lungs, and/or central vessels causes dyspnea; and that heart, lung, and neuromuscular disorders cause dyspnea. The dyspneic victims of poliomyelitis and other neurological disorders had an equally viable causality. While understanding cause is important, the missing link is mechanism, and this remains inadequately explained by work, transpulmonary pressure, oxygen debt, hypoxemia, hypercarbia, acidemia, or increased ventilation. The theory of length/tension inappropriateness, and subsequently length/length inadequacy, provided an explanation for dyspnea, but in its simple form it did not account for the dyspnea of increased ventilation in the absence of mechanical or neuromuscular defects.

III. Sensory Physiology

The emergence of interest in sensory mechanisms was an inevitable consequence of this evolution in understanding. Conscious sensation (light, sound, taste, olfaction, touch, muscular forces and movement, and presumably that of more complex sensory experiences such as discomfort with breathing) is initiated by physical stimuli which gain entry to the nervous system by acting on sensory receptors. The magnitude of the stimuli results in a graded alteration in the receptors which are transformed into a graded firing frequency in afferent nerves. The afferent nerve relays the conditions at the proximal receptors coded by firing frequency and the specific receptors stimulated to the central nervous system. Central impression of the condition of peripheral receptors is formulated; this information is interpreted in the light of experience and learning; and this process leads to conscious sensation.[28]

STIMULUS → RECEPTOR → AFFERENT NERVE → CENTRAL IMPRESSION

CENTRAL IMPRESSION → EXPERIENCE/LEARNING →
ATTENTION → CONSCIOUSNESS

The simple scheme provides the fundamental units of sensory processes. However, most sensations are compound and not discrete functions of a given receptor or sets of receptors operating alone. Compound sensations involve multiple, different types of receptors, each operating in a systematic fashion. The quality of a given sensation is related to the specific receptors stimulated, the magnitude of stimulation, and the conditions simultaneously occurring in other sets of sensory receptors activated by the same or related stimuli. Quality is multidimensional and involves the stimulation of multiple receptor types. Quantity often is unidimensional and involves a specific receptor type.

IV. Basic Sensory Neuroanatomy of Respiratory Sensation

Dyspnea reaches consciousness through the sensory infrastructure of the respiratory system. Receptors, route of afferent feedback, and central processing form the infrastructure of all respiratory sensations including dyspnea. (See Table 1.)

TABLE 1. Possible Receptors for the Sensation of Dyspnea

Vagal Receptors: irritant; stretch; J receptors
Chemoreceptors: peripheral; central
Muscular Receptors: tendon organs; muscle spindles; joint and skin
    receptors
Central Collateral Discharge: efferent copy
Upper Airway Receptors

A. Receptors

1. Pulmonary Sensory Mechanisms

There are receptors in the walls of airways, in lung parenchyma, and around capillaries. They respond to a variety of stimuli both chemical and mechanical. Afferent impulses travel by means of vagal and sympathetic pathways. These receptors have been extensively studied and reviewed in recent publications by Coleridge and Coleridge.[29] Although stimulation of these receptors modifies breathing, it is uncertain if they themselves are sentient. It seems more likely that sensation is generated by the reflex motor consequences of their stimulation. Irritation of the trachea, presumably by stimulation of vagal receptors, does produce a crude visceral sensation, but it is distinguishable from dyspnea.

2. Chemoreceptors

Peripheral and central chemoreceptors respond to hypoxemia, hypercapnia, and changes in hydrogen ion concentration, and their stimulation causes dyspnea. These receptors have been extensively studied and reviewed.[30,31] Their stimulation results in increased respiratory muscle activity and in activation of muscular and pulmonary receptors, making it difficult to isolate the sensation resulting from chemoreceptor activation alone from that generated by muscular and/or pulmonary receptors. Total neuromuscular blockade provides an opportunity to isolate chemoreceptor activity from its motor consequences. Neuromuscular blockade to the point of apnea results in an inevitable increase in chemoreceptor activity, but is not accompanied by dyspnea as shown by Campbell and colleagues.[32] The results of these studies oppose the idea that chemoreceptor activity directly results in discomfort. Dyspnea appears to be a consequence of muscular activation and not a direct consequence of chemoreceptor activity.

3. Muscular Receptors

The proprioceptive properties of muscle in general are shared by respiratory muscle. Tendon organs are mechanically stimulated by the tension developed by muscle, the tension is transduced into a neural firing frequency, and is transmitted to the central nervous system by afferent nerves, yielding a sensation of tension. Muscle spindles and joint receptors are mechanically stimulated by the extent and velocity of muscle contraction. The displacement achieved is transduced into a neural firing frequency and transmitted to the central nervous system by afferent peripheral nerves yielding a sensation of displacement.[33–36] Free nerve endings within muscle are mechanically and chemically stimulated. Following overuse of muscle, structural damage or leakage of cellular contents stimulates these receptors and yields a sensation of pain.

Man is thus capable of consciously perceiving a variety of sensations during muscular activity: tension, displacement, interrelationship of tension/displacement (impedance, resistance, elastance), and their derivatives in the time domain.[34–39] The quality of muscular sensation is determined primarily by the varying inputs from these different kinds of receptors and their interrelationships.

4. Central Collateral Discharge (Efferent Copy)

Interneurones located high in the central nervous system act as receptors that transduce the intensity of motor output to muscle. These interneurones transmit the intensity of motor command to the sensory cortex yielding a sensation of effort—the intensity of the motor command.[40-45]

5. Upper Airway Receptors

Receptors in the nose, nasopharynx, oropharynx, and larynx have been reviewed recently by Widdicombe.[46] Although these receptors have received little attention, reflexes arising within the upper airway are multiple, highly complex, and important in speech and in stabilizing the patency of the upper airway. Afferent activity travels via the trigeminal, glossopharyngeal, hypoglossal, and vagal nerves. Their stimulation can contribute to conscious sensation of irritation, pressure, and flow, but their role in sensing external respiratory loads remains controversial.

B. Respiratory Sensations

The availability of psychophysical techniques initiated an era in which the physical stimulus, sensory response, sensory receptors, and their afferent neural pathways constituted the components.[47-49]

1. The Sensation of Loaded Breathing

The sensation of loaded breathing deserves special attention because increases in mechanical loads are common to most clinical conditions in which dyspnea occurs, and because this information has shed light on basic mechanisms. Campbell et al.[50] and Bennett et al.[51] showed that humans can detect small added loads to breathing (elastic and resistive). These investigators reasoned that a change in pressure, volume, or flow alone could not explain detection because pressure, volume, and flow change during the course of normal breathing, and they are not appreciated as a change in load. They concluded that the most likely explanation was a change in the relationship between pressure and volume (elastance) and pressure and flow (resistance). Both pressure (tension) and volume (displacement) are mechanical stimuli amenable to transduction by known sensory receptors activated by respiratory muscle activity. These simple psychophysical experiments on load detection paved the way for studies on other respiratory sensations.

During the sixties, the neuroanatomy of respiratory load detection received attention with the introduction of reliable threshold detection and discrimination techniques. By comparing load detection applied at the mouth and the trachea, with and without airway anesthesia, and with and without vagal blockade in patients with complete spinal blockade at various levels, it became possible to define the neuroanatomy of load detection with classical neurophysiological techniques.

These studies showed that: (1) load detection bears a relatively fixed relationship to the magnitude of the background load[52]; (2) load detection at the mouth deteriorates in patients with airflow limitation but is similar when expressed as a fraction of background load, suggesting that upper airway receptors are unlikely to be the primary receptors[53-55]; (3) load detection is unaffected by vagal blockade[56]; (4) load detection is unaffected by local anesthesia to the airway[57]; (5) load detection is preserved as long as any respiratory muscle is capable of sustaining ventilation, as with high spinal neuromuscular blockade[58-60]; and (6) load detection is virtually abolished when the respiratory muscles are inactive (passive ventilation).[61] These studies, while refuting some of the other popular alternatives, support the concept introduced by Campbell and his colleagues of "inappropriateness."[26,27] The primary receptors, tendon organs (tension), and spindles (displacement — volume and flow) relay the afferent information and the interrelationship is centrally processed.

2. Dimensions of Respiratory Sensation

In 1970, Bakers and Tenney[62] showed that humans can directly estimate the magnitude of volume, ventilation, and respiratory pressures using open magnitude scaling. This report was followed by a variety of similar studies and established that humans can consciously perceive the magnitude of external loads,[55,63] internal loads,[64] magnitude of respiratory pressures,[65] magnitude of volume,[66-68] and magnitude of effort.[40,43,45]

These studies have been accompanied by others investigating the neurophysiological mechanism through which these sensory events were perceived. Complete agreement has not emerged yet, but the following statements represent a broad consensus. Volume changes probably are sensed through muscle spindles and joint receptors, similar to position sense in peripheral limb movement.[66-69] Tension is sensed through tendon organs. The sensation of effort is sensed by efferent copy by collateral discharge. Sherrington's[39] opposition to a separate sense of effort (sense of willed motor command) has been largely refuted; tension and effort are accepted as separate sensory events. The idea that humans can sense the intensity of the motor command to muscle in general,[35,36] and respiratory muscle in particular,[40,43,45] is reasonably accepted.

V. Assessment of Dyspnea

Having reviewed some of the basic mechanisms in the generation of respiratory sensation, we will now view these mechanisms in the context of dyspnea. The assessment of dyspnea requires first, the realization that dyspnea is a sensation; second, that sensation results from the stimulation of sensory receptors activated by the act of breathing; third, its quality depends on the conditions of stimulation in all receptor types stimulated under the conditions in which it is experienced; and fourth, basic understanding of the principles of psychophysics which are used to their greatest advantage when the intensity of stimulation of specific receptor types can be controlled and measured. Thus, knowledge of these receptors and the conditions of their stimulation are a prerequisite to fundamental understanding. However, for practical purposes we presently are limited to measuring the conditions of their stimulation (exercise, hypoxemia, hypercapnia, loaded breathing) and can make only crude approximations regarding the intensity of specific receptor stimulation.

The stimuli and receptors important in the generation of dyspnea are singled out with this background of understanding: knowledge of the common clinical and physiological conditions under which dyspnea occurs; and knowledge of a viable neurophysiological mechanism which is in agreement with the known properties of the sensory system. Hypotheses then are considered, tested using established psychophysical techniques, and refuted, modulated, or accepted based on experimental results. This approach has only recently been applied to the problem of dyspnea.

The first problem with this approach is the isolation of the stimulus or stimuli. Whereas we often measure the conditions of stimulation, e.g., the intensity of an added load or the magnitude of ventilation, these events are remote from the proximal receptors stimulated. Receptor stimulation can be crudely approximated in the following manner:

MOTOR COMMAND (Maximum Motor Command) →
TENSION (Maximum Tension) →

RATE OF DISPLACEMENT (Maximum Rate of Displacement)

Motor Command: Motor command can be approximated by expressing the activity of the muscle as a percentage of maximum achievable activity. The rationale for this approach is simple. If the activity generated with maximal effort represents recruitment of all motor units, then expressing the actual activity measured as a proportion of maximal activity gives a measurement of motor command relative to maximal, as long as the conditions of operation are the same.

Tension: Tension can be approximated by measuring pressure.

Displacement: Displacement can be approximated by measuring volume and its time derivatives (flow).

Although the approach is simple, there are problems associated with it: the conversion of tension to pressure involves complex mechanical considerations; pressure results from the recruitment of various respiratory muscles such that receptor stimulation is remote; and the velocity and extent of inspiratory muscle shortening and volume are not synonymous. Despite these problems, this approach provides an understanding of how the intensity of dyspnea varies in a number of clinical settings. The sensation of dyspnea is clarified by formally identifying how the various factors (exercise, hypercapnia, hypoxemia, neuromuscular weakness, etc.) alter the stimulation of the various sensory receptors. The roles of exercise, mechanical load, hypoxemia, hypercapnia, and acidemia readily fall into place. Dyspnea emerges as a sensory experience whose quality varies with the stimulus conditions at the various sensory receptors. The intensity of stimulation at each receptor, as well as interrelationships in time and between each receptor, determine the overall quality and intensity of dyspnea.

In the common clinical conditions under which dyspnea is experienced, the mechanical state of the respiratory system is confined to a limited number of conditions: (1) the impedance to the action of the respiratory muscles is increased; this can be sensed by the increased effort, increased inspiratory muscle tension, and the relationship between tension and displacement (inappropriateness); (2) breathing is also increased; this can be sensed by increased effort, tension, and displacement; and (3) the respiratory muscles are weak; this can be sensed by the increased effort required to sustain ventilation. The mechanical events result in the stimulation of a variety of sensory receptors, and often all three major primary receptor types are stimulated simultaneously.

Motor output to the respiratory muscles is controlled to meet the metabolic demands imposed by the varying needs for oxygen uptake, carbon dioxide output, and hydrogen ion homeostasis. The greatest demands occur during muscular activity, particularly exercise. In meeting the required ventilation, the motor output is not only dependent on metabolic demand but also on the strength and condition (perfusion and metabolic support) of the respiratory muscles. The sensory consequences are further modified by the duration, frequency, and intensity of respiratory muscle activity and the evolution of fatigue. Mechanical efficiency of the respiratory muscles, the operating conditions of the respiratory muscle (length as well as extent and velocity of contraction), the impedance imposed by the chest cage/lungs, and the efficiency of gas exchange are independent contributors to the various receptors stimulated. The interdependent interaction of these processes and their effects on sensory structures provide the background for the mechanistic evaluation of dyspnea as illustrated in Figure 1.

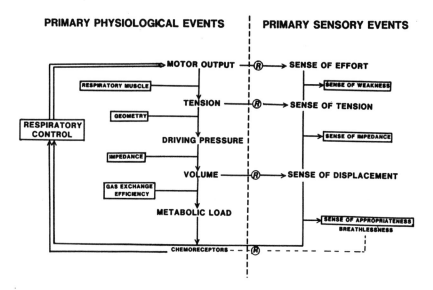

Figure 1: *Schematic representation of the interdependent interaction of physiological processes and their effects on sensory receptors.*

A. Chest Tightness

Some patients complain of a sensation of chest tightness. The circumstance under which this sensation most commonly occurs is bronchoconstriction. The lung is hyperinflated, causing the inspiratory muscles to be shortened and thus weakened; the diaphragm works at a mechanical disadvantage; inspiratory resistance and dynamic elastance are increased; ventilation frequently is increased, possibly due to irritant receptor firing, contributing to alveolar hyperventilation; and inhomeogeneous lungs contributing to dead space ventilation. This condition is associated with an inability to take a deep breath. The global quality is thus interdependent on a variety of sensory events. Individual analysis of the dimensions shows that effort is increased, tension is increased due to mechanical disadvantage and a high inspiratory impedance, impedance is increased, and inspiratory muscles are weakened. All these sensory dimensions can be individually perceived and have discrete sensory mechanisms. Their interrelationships and intensities determine the overall sensory experience.

B. Need to Breathe

Patients occasionally report that their need to breathe exceeds the current level of their breathing and that they are unable to breathe as much as they perceive is appropriate. This perceptual experience occurs in normal subjects after very short, high intensity exercise (e.g., climbing three to four flights of stairs rapidly) and is associated with a transient rise in PCO_2. Although it is tempting to suggest a link with chemoreceptor activity, the primary and secondary processing remain ill defined, and the mechanism responsible for this perception remains unknown. Acute airflow limitation is another common circumstance in which this sensory experience can occur. Effort is increased but hyperinflation commonly limits the muscular response in that the forces generated are limited by mechanical disadvantages.

C. Inappropriateness

Behavioral learning contributes additional dimensions to respiratory sensation. During the course of repeated respiratory activity, the relationships between the intensities of the primary sensations are learned. Just as individuals are aware of the amount of peripheral muscular effort involved in walking and climbing stairs, they are at least potentially aware of the respiratory muscle effort required to breathe. Although they are normally unaware of respiratory effort, this reaches consciousness *when it becomes substantial or changes*. Individuals are aware of the amount of effort, tension, and displacement expected with both peripheral and respiratory muscles under the common circumstances in which they are used. When there are changes in the effort required to generate a given ventilation, in the tension required to generate a given ventilation, in the effort required to generate a given tension, and in the ventilation required to perform a given activity, the abnormal quantitative relationships between these dimensions are readily recognized and reach consciousness. Inappropriateness between any or all of these dimensions is readily detected and contributes to respiratory sensation. Patients may sense inappropriateness at a time when discomfort is not a major concern. Inappropriateness and dyspnea are not synonymous.

VI. Summary

In summary, the causes of dyspnea have been well recognized for many years. Traditional approaches to its investigation and management have been largely confined to the identification and amelioration of these causative factors. However, dyspnea is a sensory experience and can only be fully understood with a knowledge of the sensory mechanisms. By understanding the mechanisms, approaches to both investigation and management can be improved. The quality of the sensory experience of dyspnea is formed from more than one source of information. Effort, tension, and displacement are the most important sources and account for qualitative differences. Of these sources, the intensity of dyspnea appears to be most closely related to effort.

References

1. Williams CJB. Examination of chest through functions. In: Williams CJB (ed). Pathology and Diagnosis of Diseases of Chest. 1840.
2. Pfluger E. On the causes of respiratory movements, and of dyspnea and apnea. In: West JB (ed). Translations in Respiratory Physiology. Dowden, Hutchinson, & Ross, Inc., Stroudsburg, PA, 1975; 404-434.
3. Miescher-Rusch F. Bemerkungen zur lehre von den atembewegungen. Arch Anat u Physiol Leipzig 1985; 6:355-380.
4. Haldane SJ, Smith L. 1893. In: Haldane JS, Priestley JG (eds). Respiration. Oxford, Clarendon Press, 1935.
5. Winterstein H. Die regulierung der atmung durch das blut. Zentr Physiol 1910; 24:811.
6. Meakins JM. The cause and treatment of dyspnea in cardiovascular disease. Br Med J 1923; 1:1043-1055.
7. Cullen GE, Harrison TR, Calhoun JA, et al. Regulation of dyspnea of exertion to oxygen saturation and acid-base condition of the blood. J Clin Invest 1931; 10:807.
8. Harrison TR, Harrison WG, Calhoun JA, et al. Congestive heart failure. XVII. The mechanism of dyspnea on exertion. Arch Int Med 1932; 50: 690-720.
9. Harrison TR. Failure of Circulation. Williams and Wilkins Co., Baltimore, 1935.
10. Gesell R, Moyer C. Effect of sensory nerve stimulation on costal and abdominal breathing in anaesthetized dog. Q J Exp Physiol 1935; 25:1-11.
11. Christie R. Dyspnea. Q J Med 1938; 7:421-454.
12. Means JH. Dyspnoea. Medicine 1924; 3:309-416.
13. Cournand A, Brock HJ, Rappaport L, et al. Disturbance of action of

respiratory muscles as a contributing cause of dyspnea. Arch Int Med 1936; 57:1008-26.

14. Cournand A, Richards DW. Pulmonary insufficiency. Am Rev Tuberc Pulm Dis 1941; 44:26-41.

15. Rohrer F. The physiology of respiratory movements. In: West JB (ed). Translations in Respiratory Physiology. Dowden, Hutchinson, & Ross, Inc., Stroudsburg, PA, 1975; 93-170.

16. Rahn H, Otis AB, Chadwick LE, et al. Pressure-volume diagram of the thorax and lung. Amer J Physiol 1946; 146:161-178.

17. Marshall R, McIlroy MB, Christie RV. The work of breathing in mitral stenosis. Clin Sci 1954; 13:137-146.

18. Cherniack RM, Snidal DP. The effect of obstruction to breathing on the ventilatory response to CO_2. J Clin Invest 1956; 35:1286-1290.

19. Marshall R, Stone RW, Christie RV. The relationship of dyspnoea to respiratory effort in normal subjects, mitral stenosis and emphysema. Clin Sci 1954; 13:625-631.

20. Cournand A, Richards DW, Bader RA, et al. The oxygen cost of breathing. Trans Assoc Am Physiol 1954; 67:162-173.

21. Campbell EJM, Westlake EK, Cherniack RM. Simple methods of estimating oxygen consumption and efficiency of the muscles of breathing. J Appl Physiol 1957; 11(2):303-308.

22. Campbell EJM, Westlake EK, Cherniak RM. The oxygen consumption of the respiratory muscles of young male subjects. Clin Sci 1959; 18: 55-62.

23. Bartlett RG, Brubach HF, Specht H. Oxygen cost of breathing. J Appl Physiol 1958; 14:413-424.

24. McIlroy MB. Dyspnea and the work of breathing in diseases of the heart and lungs. Prog Cardiovasc Dis 1958; 1:284-297.

25. Campbell EJM, Howell JBL. The sensation of breathlessness. Br Med Bull 1963; 19:36-40.

26. Campbell EJM. The relationship of the sensation of breathlessness to the act of breathing. In: Howell JBL, Campbell EJM (eds). Breathlessness. Oxford, Blackwell Scientific Publications, 1966; 55-64.

27. Campbell EJM. The Respiratory Muscles and the Mechanics of Breathing. Chicago, Year Book Medical Publishers, Inc., 1958.

28. Schmidt RF. Fundamentals of Sensory Physiology. New York, Springer-Verlag, 1981.

29. Coleridge HM, Coleridge JCG. Reflexes evoked from tracheobronchial tree and lungs. In: Cherniack NS, Widdicombe JG (eds). The Handbook of Physiology, Section 3: The Respiratory System. Bethesda, American Physiological Society, 1986; 395-429.

30. Fidone SJ, Gonzales C. Initiation and control of chemoreceptor activity in the carotid body. In: Cherniack NS, Widdicombe JG (eds). Handbook of Physiology, Section 3: The Respiratory System. Bethesda, American Physiological Society, 1986; 247-312.

31. Fitzgerald RS, Lahiri S. Reflex responses to chemoreceptor stimulation. In: Cherniack NS, Widdicombe JG (eds). Handbook of Physiology, Sec-

tion 3: The Respiratory System. Bethesda, American Physiological Society, 1986; 313-362.

32. Campbell EJM, Freedman S, Clark TJH, et al. The effect of muscular paralysis induced by tubocurarine on the duration and sensation of breath-holding. Clin Sci 1967; 20:223-231.
33. Gandevia SC, McCloskey DI. Joint sense, muscle sense, and their combination as position sense, measured at the distal interphalangeal joint of the middle finger. J Appl Physiol 1976; 260:387-407.
34. Matthews PBC. Evolving views on the internal operation and functional role of the muscle spindle. J Physiol 1981; 320:1-30.
35. Matthews PBC. Where does Sherrington's "Muscular Sense" originate? Muscles, joints, corollary discharge? Annu Rev Neurosci 1982; 5:189-218.
36. McCloskey DI. Kinesthetic sensibility. Physiol Rev 1978; 58:763-820.
37. Burgess PR, Wei JY, Clark FJ, et al. Signalling of kinesthetic information by peripheral sensory receptors. Annu Rev Neurosci 1982; 5:171-187.
38. Roland PE, Ladegaard-Pederson H. A quantitative analysis of sensations of tension and kinaesthesia in man. Evidence for peripherally originating muscular sense and for a sense of effort. Brain 1977; 100:671-692.
39. Sherrington CS. The muscular sense. In: Shafer EA (ed). Textbook of Physiology, Volume 2. Edinburg, Pentland, 1900; 1002-1025.
40. Campbell EJM, Gandevia SC, Killian KJ, et al. Changes in the perception of inspiratory resistive load during partial curarization. J Physiol 1980; 309:93-100.
41. Gandevia SC. The perception of motor commands or effort during muscular paralysis. Brain 1982; 105:151-195.
42. Gandevia SC, McCloskey DI. Sensation of heaviness. Brain 1977; 100: 345-354.
43. Gandevia SC, Killian KJ, Campbell EJM. The effect of respiratory muscle fatigue on respiratory sensations. Clin Sci 1981; 60:463-466.
44. Gandevia SC, McCloskey DI. Changes in motor commands, as shown by changes in perceived heaviness, during partial curarization and peripheral muscle anaesthesia in man. J Physiol 1977; 272:673-689.
45. Killian KJ, Gandevia SC, Summers E, et al. Effect of increased lung volume on perception of breathlessness, effort and tension. J Appl Physiol 1984; 57:686-691.
46. Widdicombe JG. Reflexes from the upper respiratory tract. In: Cherniack NS, Widdicombe JG (eds). Handbook of Physiology, Section 3: The Respiratory System. Bethesda, American Physiological Society, 1986; 363-394.
47. Killian KJ, Campbell EJM. Dyspnea and exercise. Annu Rev Physiol 1983; 45:465-479.
48. Killian KJ, Campbell EJM. Dyspnea. In: Roussos C, Macklem PT, (eds). The Thorax, Part B. New York, Marcel Dekker, 1985; 787-828.
49. Zechman FW Jr, Wiley RL. Afferent inputs to breathing: respiratory sensation. In: Cherniack NS, Widdicombe JG (eds). Handbook of Physiology, Section 3: The Respiratory System. Bethesda, American Physiological Society, 1986; 449-474.
50. Campbell EJM, Freedman S, Smith PS, et al. The ability of man to detect added elastic loads to breathing. Clin Sci 1961; 20:223-231.

51. Bennett ED, Jayson MIV, Rubenstein D, et al. The ability of man to detect added non-elastic loads to breathing. Clin Sci 1962; 23:155-162.
52. Wylie RL, Zechman FW Jr. Perception of added airflow resistance in humans. Respir Physiol 1966; 2:73-87.
53. Burki NK. Effects of added inspiratory loads on load detection thresholds. J Appl Physiol 1981; 50:162-164.
54. Burki NK, Mitchell K, Chaudhary BA, et al. The ability of asthmatics to detect added resistive loads. Am Rev Respir Dis 1978; 117:71-75.
55. Gottfried SB, Altose MD, Fogarty CM, et al. The perception of changes in airflow resistance in normal subjects and patients with chronic airways obstruction. Chest 1978; 73:286-288.
56. Guz A, Noble MIM, Widdicombe JG, et al. The role of vagal and glossopharyngeal afferent nerves in respiratory sensation, control of breathing and arterial pressure regulation in conscious man. Clin Sci 1966; 30:161-170.
57. Burki NK, Davenport PW, Safdar F, et al. The effects of airway anesthesia on magnitude estimation of added inspiratory resistive and elastic loads. Am Rev Respir Dis 1983; 127:2-4.
58. Eisele J, Trenchard D, Burki N, et al. The effect of chest wall block on respiratory sensation and control in man. Clin Sci 1968; 35:23-33.
59. Noble MIM, Eisele JH, Trenchard D, et al. Effect of selective peripheral nerve blocks on respiratory sensations. In: Porter R (ed). Breathing: Hering-Breuer Centenary Symposium (A Ciba Foundation Symposium). London, J & A Churchill, 1970; 233-246.
60. Zechman FW Jr., O'Neill R, Shannon R. Effect of low cervical cord lesion on detection of increased airflow resistance in man (abstract). Physiol 1967; 10:356.
61. Killian KJ, Mahutte CK, Campbell EJM. Resistive load detection during passive ventilation. Clin Sci 1980; 59:493-495.
62. Bakers JHCM, Tenney SM. The perception of some sensations associated with breathing. Respir Physiol 1970; 10:85-92.
63. Killian KJ, Mahutte CK, Campbell EJM. Magnitude scaling of externally added loads to breathing. Am Rev Respir Dis 1981; 123:12-15.
64. Burdon JGW, Juniper EF, Killian KJ, et al. Perception of breathlessness in asthma. Am Rev Resp Dis 1982; 126:825-828.
65. Stubbing DG, Ramsdale EH, Killian KJ, et al. Psychophysics of inspiratory muscle force. J Appl Physiol 1983; 54:1216-1221.
66. Stubbing DG, Killian KJ, Campbell EJM. The quantification of respiratory sensations by normal subjects. Respir Physiol 1981; 44:251-260.
67. Wolkove N, Altose MD, Kelsen SG, et al. Perception of changes in breathing in normal human subjects. J Appl Physiol 1981; 50:78-83.
68. Gliner JA, Folinsbee LJ, Horvath SM. Accuracy and precision of matching inspired lung volume. Percept Psychophys 1981; 29:511-515.
69. Salamon M, Von Euler C, Franzen O. Perception of mechanical factors in breathing. Presented at the International Symposium on Physical Work and Effort, Wenner-Gren Center, Stockholm, 1975.

Chapter 3

Clinical Measurement of Dyspnea

Donald A. Mahler and Andrew Harver

From *Dyspnea*, edited by Donald A. Mahler, M.D., © 1990, Futura Publishing Company, Inc., Mount Kisco, NY.

Measure what can be measured, make measurable what cannot be measured.

Galileo Galilei (1564-1642)

I. Introduction

Although a person may appreciate precisely his/her sensation, or feeling, of a subjective experience, words may fail to describe its exact nature. Measurement has been defined as, "The assignment of numerals to things so as to represent facts and conventions about them."[1] In the field of medicine, this process includes converting clinical descriptions of sensory experience into scientific data.[2]

The measurement of dyspnea in affected individuals is essential for several reasons. First, breathlessness is frequently an individual patient's major complaint. Second, as a symptom, breathlessness represents the sum of pathophysiological and psychological factors that collectively results in a distressing signal and frequently motivates a patient to seek medical assistance. By quantifying dyspnea, the health-care provider can assess its severity and the impact of this distressful experience on quality of life. Third, and probably most important, measurement of dyspnea is an important consideration for evaluating efficacy of treatment. At present, there is no objective evidence that any therapy, except for oxygen,[3] prolongs survival or alters the decline in lung function in chronic respiratory disorders.[4,5] Accordingly, because treatment should be directed toward improving symptoms, especially dyspnea, objective measurement of this sensation is warranted.

Can dyspnea be measured? Certainly, but only *as long as specific criteria are used*. The ability to quantify breathlessness depends on the availability of *valid, reliable,* and *sensitive* instruments to grade its severity.[6,7] These criteria are fundamental and are employed in evaluating instruments used to measure any construct.

II. Principles of Measurement

A. Measurement Scales

Four general types of measurement scales have been described:[8] nominal, ordinal, interval, and ratio. These scales provide varying degrees of quantitative information based on the extent to which they possess three attributes: degree of magnitude, intervals between adjacent units, and an absolute zero point.

Nominal scales are the simplest measurement scales because they possess none of these attributes and involve only the categorization of elements. Accordingly, a nominal scale is a simple tool for measuring the severity of dyspnea. The basic question addressed by a nominal scale is whether levels of the severity of breathlessness can be grouped in terms of specific descriptive categories of experience.

An ordinal scale ranks observations according to whether they possess more, less, or the same amount of dyspnea. Although indications of "better than," "worse than," or "equal to" are meaningful comparisons, an ordinal scale does not establish an absolute value for comparing the magnitude of difference between units on the scale.

Both interval and ratio scales offer more sophisticated approaches to the measurement of dyspnea. They possess properties of magnitude and equal intervals between units or points on the scale. In addition, ratio scales have an absolute zero point. An example of a commonly used interval scale is a thermometer for measurement of temperature in degrees centigrade. Zero on the centigrade scale does not imply the absence of heat, but rather a relative level or magnitude. However, measurement of length, weight, or degrees Kelvin is accomplished with a ratio scale in which case the computation of proportions (ratios) is meaningful.

Most clinical dyspnea scales can be considered to be between ordinal and interval levels of measurement. However, the relative merits of any instrument depend on its validity, reliability, and sensitivity (Table 1). These criteria are critical for a scale that is to be applied for clinical or research purposes.

Table 1. Definition of Terms for Principles of Measurement

Scaling—development of measurement scales.
Validity—extent to which an instrument measures what it purports to measure.
Reliability—estimate of the error component involved in the measurement of a variable.
Sensitivity—the degree to which a scale or index detects clinically important changes.

B. Validity

Validity is the extent to which an instrument measures what it purports to measure.[6] In other words, does the scale or index appear to measure the underlying trait or construct of interest? For measurement of dyspnea, no absolute criterion or standard exists.

Three basic issues should be considered in the evaluation of the validity of an instrument.[6] **Content validity** refers to the fact that a group of experts developed the instrument or tool for measuring dyspnea based on their knowledge and experience. Content validity depends on how much is known about breathlessness; however, it may be difficult to ascertain with authority. **Concurrent validity** is criterion-related, and is based on the extent to which a new scale correlates with other existing scales for measuring dyspnea. For example, a new dyspnea index would be expected to correlate (to various degrees) with previously developed scales for quantifying breathlessness. **Construct validity** relates to ". . . a hypothesis that a variety of behaviors will correlate with one another in studies of individual differences and/or will be similarly affected by experimental treatments."[6] Ideally, construct validity should be examined prospectively when an intervention or treatment is expected to strongly affect related outcomes in a predicted manner. The validity of any measure of dyspnea can be established only in a matter of degree, not in an absolute manner. Furthermore, the process of validation may be unending.

C. Reliability

A measurement instrument can be reliable without being valid; but to be valid, it must be reliable. Reliability of a scale or index concerns the estimate of the error component evident in the measurement of a variable.[6] At least three types of reliability are relevant to the measurement of dyspnea. **Test-retest reliability** concerns the variability of responses obtained from an instrument at two different points in time in individuals considered to be stable. **Inter-rater reliability** is the extent to which different observers (raters) assign similar scores for the same individual subjects with an instrument. The observers should be selected based on common experience or training and should rate dyspnea in symptomatic individuals. **Intra-rater re-**

liability relates to the consistency of scores assigned to individuals by a single observer. The usual approach to assess intra-rater reliability is for a single observer to rate a stable trait or characteristic at two different time periods in the same individuals.

D. Sensitivity

The majority of data on the measurement of dyspnea almost exclusively deals with evaluation of the symptom at a single point in time. Obviously, serial measurements of dyspnea are essential to assess change over time, especially in response to therapy.

Sensitivity denotes the degree to which a scale or index detects clinically important changes.[6,9] Demonstration of sensitivity generally depends upon improvement in dyspnea scores when therapy of *known or established* efficacy is provided, or when the use of an instrument in a clinical trial shows subsequent responsiveness to improvement in dyspnea. Furthermore, construct validity can also be established when a change in breathlessness is correlated significantly with a change in an associated variable, such as lung function or exercise performance.

A related issue is the property of the dyspnea scale or index to detect a difference, if one exists, based on appropriate numbers of subjects (power). More sensitive instruments provide greater statistical power. On the other hand, if the sensitivity of the scale is small, then an extraordinary number of subjects may be required to observe a statistically significant change in dyspnea. Such a characteristic of the scale or index would severely limit its use in clinical or research trials. Both practical experience and theoretical considerations are important to establish the sensitivity and power of clinical dyspnea instruments.

III. Clinical Rating Methods

A. Description

1. Category Scales

Fletcher[10] first published a five-point scale in 1952 that was employed by the Pneumoconiosis Research Unit (PRU) to rate the impact of dyspnea on activities relative to individuals of comparable age (Appendix A). Three years later, the PRU scale was reduced to a four-point scale for estimating severity of dyspnea by eliminating the most severe category[11] (Appendix B). Subsequently, Fletcher and colleagues[12] published a revised version of the original five-point rating system which focused on the patient's report of dyspnea while either walking distances on a level or climbing stairs (Appendix C). This questionnaire has also been referred to as the Medical Research Council (MRC) Scale because the British agency provided funding to Fletcher.[12]

In l968, Rose and Blackburn[13] developed a dyspnea questionnaire for the World Health Organization (WHO) that has been used as a part of a health insurance study (Appendix D). In 1982, the American Thoracic Society published a modification of the MRC scale[14] (Appendix E). In l986, the MRC of Great Britain incorporated three questions on activities leading to breathlessness as part of a Questionnaire on Respiratory Symptoms[15] (Appendix F).

These various scales are quite similar in content and require the patient to select from among several grades of activity the type of physical task that results in breathlessness. Although many patients are able to identify specific activities that lead to dyspnea, some others are frustrated by the limited number of choices and by the lack of clear limits between grades. Furthermore, because the categories are broad, it may be very difficult to establish an improvement in dyspnea following a therapeutic intervention.

2. Visual Analogue Scales

In l969, Aitken et al.[16] reported the use of a horizontal visual analogue scale (VAS) for quantifying sensations induced by respiratory loads. This technique, which has also been used to assess pain severity,[17] provides a more flexible approach for measuring dyspnea compared to the previously described category scales. The VAS consists of a line, usually 100 mm in length, which represents the range of severity of a symptom. A vertically oriented VAS is commonly used to assess the magnitude of dyspnea. The bottom of the scale can be described by the phrase "no breathlessness," while the top can correspond to "greatest breathlessness"[18] (Appendix G) or "shortness of breath as bad as can be."[19] The patient is asked to mark the line at a point which corresponds to his/her experience of breathlessness during a specific task or over a specific time period. In some cases, investigators have referenced the upper limit of the VAS to the level of breathlessness experienced by a patient during the stimulation of ventilation, such as by exercise or rebreathing carbon dioxide.[20] The distance from zero (the bottom of the scale in Appendix G) to the mark on the line can be measured (in millimeters) to provide a quantitative rating of dyspnea intensity.

To use these scales, instructions to the patient need to be clear and consistent. For example, responses on the VAS could be based on various activities of daily living, performance of a single task such as walking for a given time or distance, or overall activities for the past two weeks. Regardless of these conditions, the patient must receive specific and concise instructions for converting an estimate of dyspnea to a precise location on a line.

In 1978, McGavin and colleagues[21] published the oxygen-cost diagram (OCD), a specific analogue scale for measuring dyspnea (Appendix H). The OCD consists of a 100-mm line with everyday activities listed alongside the line, spaced according to the oxygen requirement associated with performing each task. The patient is instructed to mark a point on the vertical line above which he/she would become breathless. Again, the estimate is quantified by measuring the distance of the mark in millimeters above zero. Because the OCD includes various options in terms of specific activities that could elicit breathlessness, some patients need assistance or repeated instructions for marking the vertical line at an appropriate level.

3. Multidimensional Indexes

The various category and analogue scales are limited by their focus on a single dimension provoking dyspnea, i.e., magnitude of task. Consequently, multidimensional instruments have been developed to include additional components that affect the experience of breathlessness. In 1984, Mahler et al.[22] published two new indexes for rating dyspnea that included measurement of functional impairment (the degree to which activities of daily living are impaired) and magnitude of effort (the overall effort exerted to perform activities), in addition to magnitude of task, that provoked difficult breathing. The Baseline Dyspnea Index (BDI) was developed to rate the severity of dyspnea at a single point in time, and the Transition Dyspnea Index (TDI) was devised to measure changes from a baseline condition (Appendix I). At the initial or baseline evaluation, the patient's status is rated by an observer from 0 (severe) to 4 (unimpaired) for each of the three categories. The ratings from each category are added together to form a baseline focal score (range, 0 to 12). The lower the score, the worse the dyspnea. Transitions, or changes, in a patient's status are compared to the baseline state through ratings obtained on a seven-point scale for each category. Scores range from −3 (major deterioration) to +3 (major improvement). The ratings on each of the categories are summed to form a transition focal score (range, −9 to +9).

Scores for the baseline and transition ratings of dyspnea are obtained through an interview conducted by an observer (physician, nurse, or technician) experienced in obtaining a clinical history for respiratory disease. For each category, the interviewer asks open-ended questions about the patient's experience of breathlessness, while at the same time focuses on specific criteria for evaluating the severity or intensity of breathlessness. Based on the patient's responses, the observer can grade the degree of impairment related to dyspnea. This process enables the interviewer to grade an individual's dyspnea from responses to standard questions asked of a patient.

In 1986, Stoller et al.[23] modified the BDI by dividing the category of functional impairment into work and home components, and separated "threshold" and "maximum" tasks for the categories of magnitude of task and effort (Appendix J). Further instructions also were provided for assigning a composite functional score.

One year later, Guyatt and colleagues[24] published the Chronic Respiratory Questionnaire (CRQ) to assess quality of life in patients with chronic lung disease (Appendix K). Dyspnea is one of four dimensions measured in the CRQ. To evaluate dyspnea, each patient is asked to select the five most bothersome activities that elicited breathlessness during the last two weeks. A list of 26 activities is then read to the patient who responds whether shortness of breath occurred with any activity. After the patient determines the five most important activities affecting daily life, the severity of breathlessness is determined using a 1 ("extremely short of breath") to 7 ("not at all short of breath") scale. These scores are added to obtain an overall CRQ dyspnea score (range, 5 to 35). The authors provide, upon request, specific instructions for use of the CRQ.[24]

B. Validity

Most clinical rating methods of dyspnea possess content validity. In other words, the various scales and indexes were developed by "a group of experts" from the fields of respiratory medicine and physiology.

Concurrent validity has been examined by comparing scores for breathlessness in the same symptomatic patients using different rating methods. For example, Guyatt and colleagues[25] found that the WHO scale, the OCD, and the BDI were significantly related ($r = 0.59$ to 0.73) in 43 patients (25 with respiratory disease and 18 with cardiac disease). Stoller et al.[23] studied 32 patients with stable chronic obstructive pulmonary disease (COPD) and found that the modified BDI correlated significantly ($r_s = -0.62$; $p < 0.001$) with the PRU score. In addition, the authors reported that the modified BDI appeared to be "more sensitive" than the PRU because it identified different degrees of dyspnea among patients with identical PRU scores. Relatively little agreement among the three categories for the modified BDI was found, suggesting that each of the components made a distinct contribution to the clinical measurement of dyspnea. Mahler and Wells[26] reported significant correlations among the scores from the modified MRC, OCD, and BDI in 153 patients with various respiratory diseases (Figure 1). Mahler et al.[27] also found that clinical ratings of breath-

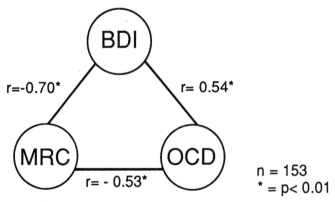

Figure 1: *Correlations among three clinical methods for rating dyspnea in 153 patients with various respiratory diseases. MRC = modified Medical Research Council scale; OCD = oxygen-cost diagram; BDI = baseline dyspnea index. (Results summarized from Mahler DA, Wells CK. Evaluation of clinical methods for rating dyspnea. Chest 1988; 93:580-586, with permission.)*

Table 2. Sensitivity of Clinical Methods for Rating Dyspnea

Rating Method	t value	p value
TDI	6.36	0.001
CRQ dyspnea	5.97	0.001
Modified MRC	1.12	0.28
OCD	1.05	0.31

Differences before and after a pulmonary rehabilitation program. TDI = Transition dyspnea index; CRQ = Chronic respiratory questionnaire; MRC = Medical Research Council; OCD = Oxygen-cost diagram.
Results summarized from Guyatt GH, Berman LB, Townshend M, et al. A measure of quality of life for clinical trials in chronic lung disease. Thorax 1987; 42:773–778.

lessness were highly interrelated (MRC vs. OCD, $r_s = -0.80$; MRC vs. BDI, $r_s = -0.87$; and OCD vs. BDI, $r_s = 0.70$; $p < 0.001$ for all comparisons) in 20 patients with interstitial lung disease (ILD). Gift[19] demonstrated a significant correlation between dyspnea scores on a vertical VAS and a horizontal VAS ($r = 0.97$) in 16 asthmatic subjects. These overall findings demonstrate that estimates of dyspnea obtained with different clinical rating methods are significantly related. Such correlations provide evidence for concurrent validity among the instruments.

Several studies have evaluated construct validity of clinical dyspnea scales. Guyatt et al.[24] evaluated changes in different dyspnea scales after a pulmonary rehabilitation program (Table 2). The TDI and CRQ dyspnea dimension showed comparable improvements in breathlessness between baseline (before rehabilitation) and follow-up (after rehabilitation), whereas there was no significant change in dyspnea ratings on either the modified MRC scale or OCD.[24] Gift[19] reported construct validity for the vertical VAS in patients with asthma and COPD using the contrasted-groups approach with repeated measures. Further support for construct validity of clinical dyspnea scales is provided in two clinical trials. Murciano et al.[28] demonstrated that improvement in dyspnea (on a VAS) with sustained-release theophylline was correlated significantly with an increase in respiratory muscle function in 60 patients with COPD. Harver et al.[29] found significant relationships between changes in inspiratory muscle strength and maximal voluntary ventilation with changes in magnitude of task and effort components of the BDI after targeted inspiratory muscle training in an experimental group of 10 COPD patients. These collective results suggest that the VAS[19] and two multidimensional scales[22,24] exhibit construct validity based on corresponding changes in ratings of dyspnea.

C. Reliability

Guyatt and associates[25] evaluated test-retest reliability for various clinical dyspnea rating methods in 43 patients at six different times with two-week intervals. Correlation coefficients and kappa values were significant ($p < 0.001$) among scores for the WHO dyspnea questionnaire, OCD, and BDI at six different visits.[25]

Scores from scales or indexes which are graded by an interviewer and not by the individual patient raise the critical question of inter-rater agreement. For the PRU dyspnea scale, Schilling et al.[11] reported relatively poor agreement between two different observers using the four question scale among both control subjects and cotton workers. However, Mahler et al.[22,26,30] found that both percentage agreement and the weighted kappa value, which accounts for disparities in ranks and adjusts for the amount of agreement that might occur by chance alone, showed substantial congruence between different observers for BDI scores in patients with various respiratory disorders. The OCD also showed good agreement on repeated use by the same individual patients.[26]

These overall results indicate that several of the clinical rating methods provide acceptable levels of test-retest and inter-rater reliability. Additional studies are needed to expand these findings and to evaluate intra-rater characteristics.

D. Sensitivity

Although the MRC scale has been used extensively for epidemiologic studies, diagnostic evaluation, and clinical trials, it appears to be too coarse to demonstrate reliable changes in breathlessness following an intervention.[22,24,26,31] Serial measurements of dyspnea using a VAS might be effective for showing change within a single patient, but this method may not be appropriate for comparing dyspnea in different patients nor may it be satisfactory for comparing the conditions of groups of patients. Nevertheless, the VAS has been applied in several clinical studies and has demonstrated improvement in dyspnea after various interventions.[28,32–35]

Two different multidimensional scales have been developed to quantify changes from a baseline state.[22,24] Each of these techniques utilizes specific criteria for determining interval changes in dyspnea. Mahler and colleagues[22] devised the TDI (Appendix I) to determine transitions or changes from a baseline state. Guyatt et al.[24] constructed the CRQ which included dyspnea as one of the four dimensions affecting quality of life (Appendix K). Both instruments have been used in clinical trials to demonstrate reductions in dyspnea with bronchodilator therapy in patients with COPD.[36,37] An additional study evaluating targeted inspiratory muscle training in COPD patients has demonstrated improvement in dyspnea using the BDI and TDI.[29]

Therefore, the VAS[18,19] as well as the two multidimensional scales[22,24] appear to be sensitive instruments which demonstrate expected changes in dyspnea as a result of specific therapy.

E. Relationship with Physiological Function

In 1842, Beau and Maissiat[38] described a "respiratory pulse" based on vigorous contraction of the scalene and sternocleidomastoid muscles in severe COPD. This observation was previously reported as an "index of dyspnea."[38,39] Over the past decade, several studies have examined correlations among dyspnea scores and various measures of respiratory and exercise function.

1. Respiratory Function

Dyspnea scores generally are related, albeit modestly, to measures of lung function in symptomatic patients with obstructive airway disease. Mahler et al.[22] found that the BDI was significantly related to both FEV_1 ($r=0.41$; $p=0.01$) and FVC ($r=0.56$; $p < 0.001$) in 38 patients with COPD (Figure 2). Stoller and coinvestigators[23] also

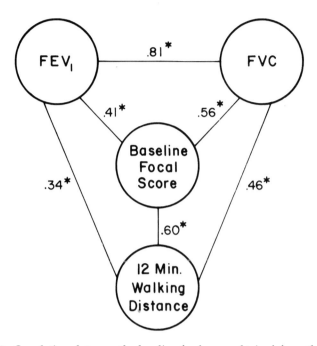

Figure 2: *Correlations between the baseline focal score obtained from the Baseline Dyspnea Index (BDI) and forced expiratory volume in one second (FEV₁), forced vital capacity (FVC), and 12-minute walking distance (12MW) in 38 patients with chronic obstructive pulmonary disease. (From Mahler DA, Weinberg DH, Wells CK, et al. The measurement of dyspnea: contents, interobserver agreement, and physiologic correlates of two new clinical indexes. Chest 1984; 85:751-758, with permission.)*

observed significant correlations between dyspnea ratings (modified BDI and the PRU) and FEV_1, FVC, and transdiaphragmatic pressure (Pdi) in COPD patients. However, neither clinical method was significantly related to arterial oxygen tension at rest ($r = 0.07$ and -0.20, respectively).[23] Mahler and colleagues[30] reported that the modified MRC scale, OCD, and BDI each correlated reliably with FVC ($r = 0.43$ to 0.49; $p < 0.05$), but only the modified MRC scale and BDI were significantly related to FEV_1 ($r = 0.44$ and 0.46, respectively; $p < 0.05$) in 24 patients with obstructive airway disease (asthma, COPD, and cystic fibrosis). Analyses conducted in 153 patients with various respiratory disorders showed that clinical ratings of breathlessness correlated significantly not only with spirometric values but also with respiratory muscle strength[26] (Figure 3). Gift[19] observed significant correlation between dyspnea scores on the vertical VAS and peak flow ($r = 0.85$) in 16 asthmatic patients.

Significant correlations have also been reported for dyspnea ratings and respiratory function in patients with interstitial lung disease (ILD). Turner-Warwick et al.[40] examined 220 patients with ILD and found that the severity of dyspnea (1–4 grade scale) was significantly

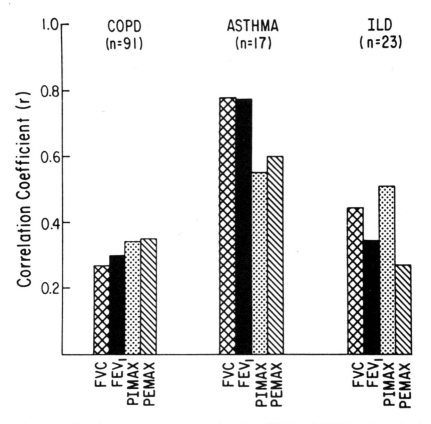

Figure 3: *Correlations among spirometric values (FVC and FEV_1) and maximal inspiratory (PIMAX) and expiratory (PEMAX) mouth pressures for three major categories: chronic obstructive pulmonary disease (COPD), asthma, and interstitial lung disease (ILD). (From Mahler DA, Wells CK. Evaluation of clinical methods for rating dyspnea. Chest 1988; 93:580-586, with permission.)*

related to both FEV_1 (p < 0.001) and FVC (p < 0.003). Mahler and colleagues[27] reported that single-breath diffusing capacity (D_LCO) was the only resting physiological parameter examined that correlated with breathlessness ($r_s = 0.59$; p < 0.05 between D_LCO and BDI) in 20 patients with ILD.

However, other studies have shown that dyspnea scores do not always correlate with measures of lung function. Mier-Jedrzejowicz et al.[41] found no correlation between dyspnea on the MRC scale and Pdi in 30 patients with weakness of the diaphragm muscle. Also, Wolkove and colleagues[42] reported that dyspnea at rest, as measured on the modified Borg scale (range, 0 to 10), was not significantly related to pre- or postbronchodilator FVC or FEV_1 in 93 patients with COPD.

2. Exercise Function

In general, a modest relationship exists between the rated severity of dyspnea and exercise capacity in symptomatic individuals. McGavin and colleagues[21] showed that the magnitude of breathlessness (grades 1 to 5) was related to the distance walked in 12 minutes (12 MW) in patients with respiratory disease. Furthermore, the OCD was significantly correlated with 12 MW ($r = 0.60$; p < 0.01).[21] Guyatt et al.[25] demonstrated that the WHO scale, OCD, and BDI were significantly correlated with six-minute walking distance ($r_s = 0.50$ to 0.59; p = 0.001 for all comparisons) in 43 patients with cardiac or respiratory disease, but that the clinical dyspnea scales were not significantly related to exercise time until exhaustion on the cycle ergometer. Stoller and colleagues[23] noted that the PRU scale, but not the modified BDI, correlated significantly with 12 MW in 32 COPD patients, 19 of whom were inpatients participating in a pulmonary rehabilitation program.

In 1971, Jones et al.[43] observed that dyspnea scores on the MRC scale generally were related to maximal power production on the cycle ergometer in patients with chronic airway obstruction (Figure 4). Subsequently, Mahler and Harver[44] examined the value of different resting variables (age, BDI, spirometry, respiratory muscle strength, diffusing capacity, and oxygen saturation) for predicting peak oxygen consumption ($\dot{V}O_2$). They reported that FEV_1, age, and

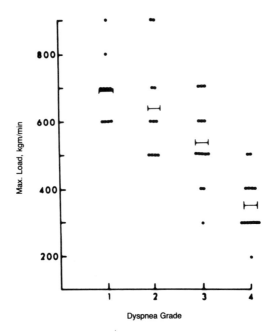

Figure 4: *Individual values for severity of breathlessness and maximal work performance on the cycle ergometer in 50 patients with chronic airflow obstruction. (From Jones NL, Jones G, Edwards RHT. Exercise tolerance in chronic airway obstruction. Am Rev Respir Dis 1971; 103:477-491, with permission.)*

the BDI score were significant and independent predictors of peak $\dot{V}O_2$ measured on the cycle ergometer in 40 symptomatic patients with obstructive airway disease. The multiple regression equation was:[44]

$$\text{peak } \dot{V}O_2 \text{ (mL/kg/min)} = 5.5 \text{ (FEV}_1) -0.3 \text{ (age)} +$$
$$0.8 \text{ (BDI)} + 19.3; \text{ SEE} = 4.2 \text{ mL/kg/min; } R^2 = 79\%.$$

The relationship between BDI scores and peak $\dot{V}O_2$ for this group is illustrated in Figure 5.

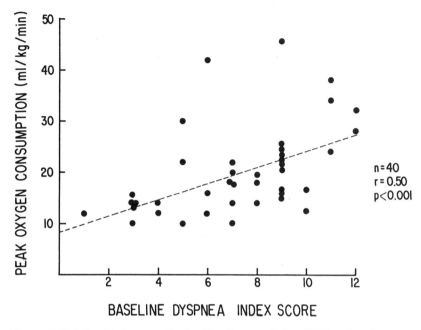

Figure 5: *Relationship between the Baseline Dyspnea Index (BDI) and peak oxygen consumption (V̇O₂) in 40 patients with symptomatic obstructive airway disease. (Data obtained from Mahler DA, Harver A. Prediction of peak oxygen consumption in obstructive airway disease. Med Sci Sports Exercise 1988; 20:574-578.)*

Mahler et al.[27] observed that clinical ratings of dyspnea (MRC, OCD, and BDI) also were related significantly to peak $\dot{V}O_2$ in patients with ILD. Furthermore, exercise gas exchange was inversely correlated with BDI scores in the ILD patients ($r_s = -0.49$; $p < 0.05$).

V. Exercise Ratings

A. Description

One of the earliest attempts to examine the experience of breathlessness was to analyze the balance between ventilatory demand and ventilatory capacity.[45] This approach relates exercise ventilation ($\dot{V}_E$) to maximal voluntary ventilation (MVV). The "dyspnea index" was devised as the $\dot{V}_E$max/MVV ratio; it was suggested that the percent of an individual's ventilatory capacity used during exercise indicated the severity of dyspnea.[46,47] When the "dyspnea index" exceeded 50%, shortness of breath was invariably present; however, many exceptions were noted.[48] Similarly, Warring[49] suggested that the ratio of walking ventilation (WV)/maximal breathing capacity (MBC), which is the same as MVV, was related to the severity of dyspnea (Figure 6). Warring[49] reported that if the WV/MBC ratio was less than 30%, the patient was not usually dyspneic. Presently, the $\dot{V}_E$/MVV ratio is predominantly used to evaluate the ventilatory reserve during exercise rather than as an estimate of dyspnea.

Exercise testing in the laboratory can simulate various physical activities of an individual that may lead to breathlessness. Such testing provides an opportunity to quantify dyspnea in a controlled setting and to elucidate the pathophysiological mechanisms that contribute to difficult or labored breathing[50] (see Chapter 6). The exercise test may involve walking in a hospital corridor for six or twelve minutes, cycle ergometry, arm ergometry, or treadmill walking. Generally, both cardiac and respiratory responses are measured during exercise. The usual parameters of cardiac function include heart rate and systemic blood pressure; the usual parameters of respiratory function include minute ventilation ($\dot{V}_E$), frequency of respiration (f_R), and tidal volume (V_T). Metabolic parameters include oxygen consumption ($\dot{V}O_2$) and carbon dioxide production ($\dot{V}CO_2$).

The patient's estimate of the severity of breathlessness during exercise is useful for several reasons. First, the intensity of dyspnea can be quantified in a standard manner. Second, the various stimuli contributing to dyspnea may be evaluated and possibly identified. Third, this information may be useful for evaluating responses to therapy.

The most widely used instruments for measuring dyspnea during exercise are the Borg category scale and the visual analogue scale. Certainly, other approaches also can be used, including open magnitude scaling and cross-modality matching (see Chapter 1).

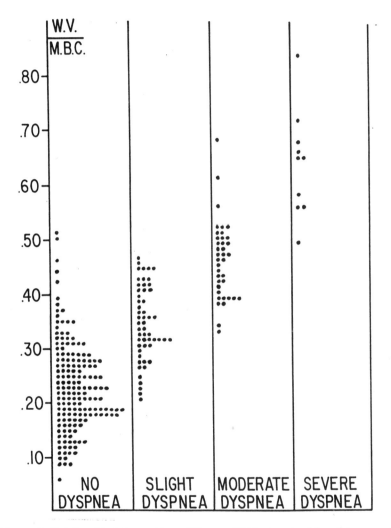

Figure 6: *Relationship between the walking ventilation/maximal breathing capacity (also called maximal voluntary ventilation) ratio and severity of dyspnea in patients with pulmonary tuberculosis. (From Warring FC Jr. Ventilatory function. Am Rev Tuberc 1945; 51:432-454, with permission.)*

1. Borg Category Scale (Appendix L)

In 1970, Borg[51] described a scale ranging from 6 to 20 for use in rating perceived exertion during a standard exercise test. The scale was modified by Borg to a simpler category scale (range, 0 to 10) with verbal expressions of severity anchored to specific numbers.[52] The non-linear spacing of expressions suggests ratio properties of sensation intensities despite constraining the full perceptual range to numbers ranging between 0 to 10. Killian and colleagues[53–57] have described extensively the use of the Borg scale for measuring dyspnea during exercise.

Specific instructions should be provided to individuals for using the Borg category scale. For example, various investigators have asked subjects to rate or estimate different respiratory sensations during exercise testing, including the "magnitude or severity of breathlessness,"[56,57] a "feeling of an uncomfortable need to breathe,"[58] and "sense of effort required to breathe."[59] For practical purposes, the numbers and descriptive phrases of the Borg scale should be large and easy to read. One approach is to hold the scale in front of the exercising individual and ask the person to point to the number which corresponds to his/her sensation of breathlessness at specific times. The person recording the rating should say the number out loud to confirm the subject's selection.

2. Visual analogue scale (Appendix G)

The VAS limits ratings of the perceived magnitude of dyspnea to the distance on a vertical or horizontal line, usually 100 mm in length. Generally, descriptive phrases for the extreme magnitudes are anchored on the VAS. For the sensation of dyspnea, zero mm (one extreme of the line) could represent "not at all breathless"[60–62] and the other extreme of the line could represent "very breathless,"[61] or "extremely breathless."[62] Stark et al.[61] referenced the top score on the VAS for each patient to the experience elicited by a standard stress greater in severity than that expected to occur during a subsequent rating period.

The VAS can be displayed on a screen positioned in front of the subject. At specific time periods, the exercising subject is asked to rate the severity of breathlessness by using a finger control to position a mark on the VAS. After the distance from the baseline is measured, the mark on the VAS can be reset to "not at all breathless."

The VAS should not be used to compare different individuals or groups. The reason for this is the anchors for extreme magnitudes are quite different in various individuals.

B. Validity

One of the basic questions concerning validity is, "What is the 'stimulus' for dyspnea during exercise?" As described in Chapter 2 of this book, the exact mechanisms subserving the sensation of breathlessness have not been completely elucidated. One approach to examine sensory-perceptual correlates of breathlessness during exercise is to apply psychophysical principles to the analysis of various stimulus-response relationships. Exercise is a physical stress which results in both physiological and psychological responses, and investigators have attempted to relate specific physiological variables, singly or in combination, to the perception of breathlessness.

The measurement of breathlessness during exercise can be examined relative to the workload, the specific physiological responses, or the combinations of responses. Power production or $\dot{V}O_2$ levels obtained during exercise have been used as independent variables to assess the intensity of dyspnea during work.[55-57,62] An example demonstrating the relationship between $\dot{V}O_2$ and Borg ratings of breathlessness during exercise is shown in Figure 7.

Numerous investigators have selected $\dot{V}_E$ as the physiological "stimulus" for evaluating ratings of dyspnea.[58-65] Exercise $\dot{V}_E$ has been used because it represents the total output of the respiratory system and it correlates significantly with dyspnea ratings.[56-65] For example, Lane et al.[64] applied resistive loading during exercise to 18 healthy subjects and found that inspired minute ventilation was a significant predictor of "uncomfortable need to breathe" on the VAS, but that the correlation coefficient (r) was only 0.29 among 648 observations. On the other hand, Silverman and colleagues[59] noted that the "perceived sense of effort in breathing" during exercise correlated closely with $\dot{V}_E$ ($r = 0.97$) in six patients with COPD.

El-Manshawi et al.[56] and LeBlanc et al.[57] have investigated the relationships among multiple physiological variables measured during exercise and the intensity of breathlessness obtained on the Borg

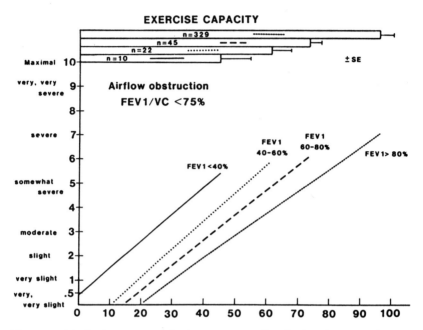

Figure 7: *Maximal oxygen uptake (as percent predicted) plotted against the Borg rating of breathlessness in normal subjects and patients with varying severity of airflow obstruction. (From Killian KJ. The objective measurement of breathlessness. Chest 1985; 88[suppl]:84S-90S, with permission.)*

category scale. LeBlanc and colleagues[57] found that the perception of breathlessness was described by the following multiple linear regression equation for 20 subjects (2 normals and 18 patients):

$$\text{Breathlessness} = 3.0 \, (P_{PL}/MIP) + 1.2 \, (\dot{V}_I) + 4.5 \, (V_T/FVC) + 0.13 \, (f_R) + 5.6 \, (T_I/T_{TOT}) - 6.2,$$

where P_{PL} is pleural pressure; MIP is maximal inspiratory pressure measured at the mouth at rest; $\dot{V}_I$ is peak inspired flow; V_T is tidal volume; FVC is forced vital capacity measured at rest; f_R is frequency of breathing; T_I is inspiratory time; and T_{TOT} is total respiratory time per breath. These variables accounted for 69% of the variance in the ratings of breathlessness. Although these data suggest possible physiological stimuli, any attempt to apply these results to clinical practice requires placement of an esophageal balloon to estimate the pleural pressure. This is not performed routinely in most cardiopulmonary exercise laboratories.

Mahler et al.[66] have evaluated the predictive value of various physiological parameters for the perception of breathlessness during cycle ergometry in patients with asthma. The Borg rating of breathlessness was used as the dependent variable. Nine independent variables were examined: $\dot{V}_E$; $\dot{V}O_2$; peak inspiratory mouth pressure (Pm); peak V_I; V_T; f_R; T_I/T_{TOT}; peak inspiratory Pm/PIMAX; and V_T/FVC. Multiple linear regression analysis relating the physiological variables to the Borg rating of breathlessness was highly significant (model F = 43.4; p < 0.0001). A backward elimination procedure selected the strongest predictors for the Borg rating of dyspnea: $\dot{V}_I$ (p = 0.0005); V_T/FVC (p = 0.0009); f_R (p = 0.0001); and Pm (p = 0.0001). These four variables explained 63% of the variance in the rating of dyspnea. Although $\dot{V}_E$, as a single independent variable, was correlated significantly with the rating of breathlessness (r = 0.67; p = 0.0001), it did not contribute significantly as an independent predictor (p = 0.84). This latter finding may be due to the fact that the individual predictor variables ($\dot{V}_I$, V_T/FVC, f_R, and Pm) are major components which determine $\dot{V}_E$.

Neither concurrent nor construct validity has been established for the use of exercise testing for measuring dyspnea in symptomatic patients. However, Adams et al.[62] examined the intensity of breathlessness resulting from hypercapnia, hypoxia, or exercise in normal subjects using the VAS and ratio magnitude estimation. Wilson and Jones[58] compared the VAS and Borg scale for measuring dyspnea during exercise in 10 normal individuals. They found that the VAS was used over a wider range than the Borg scale.

At present, the "stimulus," or combination of stimuli for evaluating the sensation of dyspnea during exercise remains obscure. Accordingly, measuring breathlessness during exercise requires careful selection of one or more physiological variables, including work itself. This choice must then be shown to fulfill both reliability and sensitivity criteria for measurement.

C. Reliability

Test-retest reliability of dyspnea ratings during exercise primarily have been examined in relation to the corresponding $\dot{V}_E$. Wilson and

Jones,[58] Stark et al.,[60,61] and Adams et al.[62] evaluated breathlessness ratings in *healthy subjects* on a VAS during treadmill exercise or cycle ergometry at repeated intervals, one day to six weeks apart. These investigators reported significant correlations between $\dot{V}_E$-VAS responses at different test periods. Wilson and Jones[58] observed that the slopes of the VAS-$\dot{V}_E$ and Borg score-$\dot{V}_E$ relationships were greater on the second day of testing than on the initial test. In addition, Stark et al.[60] described "adequate reproducibility" of $\dot{V}_E$-VAS responses in three of five patients with COPD during walking on a treadmill. Silverman and colleagues[59] found that the perceived "sense of effort in breathing" was "highly reproducible" during repeat cycle ergometry in six subjects with COPD. The relevance, however, of these results is unclear because these investigators did not address the primary question of whether the $\dot{V}_E$-VAS or $\dot{V}_E$-Borg relationship was valid for measurement of breathlessness ratings during exercise.

Mahler and colleagues[66] examined the test-retest reliability of dyspnea ratings at two different visits one week apart in 15 asthmatic patients. The individual slopes for three of the four predictor variables and Borg ratings were significantly correlated: $\dot{V}_I$-Borg ($r=0.92$; $p=0.0001$), Pm-Borg ($r=0.79$; $p=0.0005$), and f_R-Borg ($r=0.87$; $p=0.0001$). However, the slopes for V_T/FVC-Borg relationship at the two visits were not significantly related ($r=0.37$; $p=0.18$). Correlations for individual intercepts were significant for $\dot{V}_I$-Borg ($r=0.77$; $p=0.0008$), Pm-Borg ($r=0.57$; $p=0.03$), f_R-Borg ($r=0.75$; $p=0.001$), and V_T/FVC-Borg ($r=0.62$; $p=0.01$). The Borg rating of dyspnea at 50% and 100% of peak work capacity (Wcap) was also reliable between the two visits ($r=0.56$; $p=0.03$ and $r=0.99$; $p=0.0001$, respectively).

D. Sensitivity

Various investigators have evaluated the possible benefits of different therapy on the intensity of dyspnea during exercise in patients. These studies have specifically examined the relationship between exercise $\dot{V}_E$ and the corresponding dyspnea rating to assess medications[61,67,68] or supplemental oxygen.[34,69,70] Once again, the question of the validity of this approach has yet to be convincingly established. Stark et al.[61] estimated the sensitivity of dyspnea ratings on the VAS relative to $\dot{V}_E$ during treadmill walking in five patients with asthma. Responses were evaluated 20 to 30 minutes after a placebo aerosol and 20 to 30 minutes after a bronchodilator aerosol in a non-randomized protocol on the same day. Although the authors state that ". . . the test was sensitive enough to detect an effective treatment," examination of the results indicate that appropriate statistical analyses were not performed.

Guyatt et al.[37] also used the VAS to quantify dyspnea after different bronchodilators (albuterol metered-dose inhaler and sustained-release theophylline) in COPD patients. The dyspnea ratings were obtained after patients completed a six-minute walking test. There was significant improvement in the VAS dyspnea ratings after each type of therapy.[37]

The Borg category scale also has been used to evaluate dyspnea during exercise tests as a result of therapy. Light et al.[68] reported that Borg scores of dyspnea were significantly lower at the highest equivalent workload during cycle ergometry after a single dose of oral morphine compared to placebo. Mahler et al.[71] examined the criterion of sensitivity during progressive incremental exercise in asthmatic patients. Acute changes in lung function were induced by random administration of inhaled metaproterenol (a bronchodilator) or inhaled methacholine (a bronchoconstrictor) one week apart. There was an increase of $14 \pm 11\%$ in FEV_1 after the bronchodilator and a decrease of $36 \pm 11\%$ in FEV_1 after the bronchoconstrictor prior to exercise. Analysis of variance showed significant increases in Borg ratings of dyspnea at 50% and 100% of peak Wcap on the cycle ergometer with methacholine compared to both baseline and bronchidilator conditions. In contrast, there were no significant differences in slopes or intercepts for select physiological variables ($\dot{V}_I$, Pm, f_R, and V_T/FVC) and Borg ratings of breathlessness.[71]

V. Summary

Both clinical rating methods and exercise ratings have been used to measure dyspnea in symptomatic patients. The measurement process is based, in part, on the principles of psychophysics (see Chapter 1) despite the uncertainty of the "stimulus" for dyspnea (see Chapter 2). Based on results of comparative studies in different patient populations, both of these approaches appear to provide unique and distinct information about dyspnea.[27,30,64,72] These findings are not surprising because the conditions and instructions for measurement of the sensation of breathlessness are different for each technique.

Which approach for measuring dyspnea should be used? The answer to this question depends entirely upon the purpose or intent of measurement. Based on the information reviewed in this chapter, the following recommendations can be made. Clinical rating methods appear most appropriate for evaluating the impact of dyspnea on a patient's daily activities and for assessing the clinical response to therapy. Of the available clinical methods for quantifying dyspnea (Appendices A-K), the VAS[18,19] and the multidimensional rating tools[22,24] generally fulfill the criteria of validity, reliability, and sensitivity. However, additional studies are needed to further evaluate these instruments.

Measurement of dyspnea during exercise testing provides an opportunity to standardize an activity which provokes breathlessness in patients. Furthermore, numerous physiological variables can be recorded and related to the corresponding ratings of dyspnea. However, at the present time, more investigations are necessary to determine the following: the most appropriate exercise "stimulus" for analyzing the intensity of breathlessness; the reliability of ratings during exercise; and sensitivity in response to specific therapy. Accordingly, exercise testing can not be recommended for routine measurement of dyspnea until further information on these criteria are available.

Finally, psychophysical testing appears useful for investigating the perceptual sensation of breathlessness in relation to standard physical stimuli or physiological conditions *in the laboratory*. Although the principles of psychophysics are applied to quantify the intensity of dyspnea for both clinical rating methods and exercise ratings, neither threshold detection nor magnitude estimation seem appropriate for the clinical measurement of dyspnea (see Chapter 1).

Appendices

APPENDIX A

Intitial Pneumoconiosis Research Unit Dyspnea Questionnaire

Grade 1: Is the patient's breath as good as that of other men of his own age and build at work, on walking, and on climbing hills or stairs?

Grade 2: Is the patient able to walk with normal men of own age and build on the level but unable to keep up on hills or stairs?

Grade 3: Is the patient unable to keep up with normal men on the level, but able to walk about a mile or more at his own speed?

Grade 4: Is the patient unable to walk more than about 100 yards on the level without a rest?

Grade 5: Is the patient breathless on talking or undressing, or unable to leave his house because of breathlessness?

From Fletcher CM. The clinical diagnosis of pulmonary emphysema—an experimental study. Proc R Soc Med 1952; 45:577–584, with permission.

APPENDIX B

Revised Pneumoconiosis Research Unit Dyspnea Questionnaire

Grade 1: Is your breathing as good as that of normal men of your own age and build on climbing hills or stairs?

Grade 2: Are you able to keep up with normal men on the level but unable to keep up on hills and stairs?

Grade 3: Are you unable to keep up with normal men of the level but able to walk a mile or more at own speed without stopping?

Grade 4: Are you unable to walk about half a mile but able to walk about a hundred yards without stopping?

From Schilling RSF, Hughes JPW, Dingwall-Fordyce I. Disagreement between observers in an epidemiological study of respiratory disease. Br Med J 1955; 1:65–68, with permission.

APPENDIX C
Breathlessness Questionnaire

Grade 1: Are you ever troubled by breathlessness except on strenuous exertion? ( )

Grade 2: (If yes.) Are you short of breath when hurrying on the level or walking up a slight hill? ( )

Grade 3: (If yes.) Do you have to walk slower than most people on the level? Do you have to stop after a mile or so (or after ½ hours) on the level at your own pace? ( )

Grade 4: (If yes to either.) Do you have to stop for breath after walking about 100 yards (or after a few minutes) on the level? ( )

Grade 5: (If yes.) Are you too breathless to leave the house, or breathless after undressing? ( )

From Fletcher CM, Elmes PC, Wood CH. The significance of respiratory symptoms and the diagnosis of chronic bronchitis in a working population. Br Med J 1959; 2: 257–266, with permission.

APPENDIX D
Dyspnoea Questionnnaire
(for administration by an interviewer)

1. Are you troubled by shortness of breath when hurrying on level ground or walking up a slight hill? . . . . ☐ Yes ☐ No
   If "No", stop here. If "Yes", proceed to next question.

2. Do you get short of breath walking with other people of your own age on level ground? . . . . ☐ Yes ☐ No
   If "No", stop here. If "Yes", proceed to next question.

3. Do you have to stop for breath when walking at your own pace on level ground? ☐ Yes ☐ No
   If "No", stop here. If "Yes", proceed to next question.

4. Are you short of breath on washing or dressing? ☐ Yes ☐No

*   *
*

On the basis of the subject's answers, dyspnoea may be graded as follows:

Q.1:   "Yes" } = Grade 1
Q.2–4: "No"

Q.1–2: "Yes" } = Grade 2
Q.3–4: "No"

Q.1–3: "Yes" } = Grade 3
Q.4:   "No"

Q.1–4: "Yes" = Grade 4

From Rose GA, Blackburn H, Gillum RF, et al. Cardiovascular Survey Methods, 2nd Edition. Geneva, World Health Organization, 1982; 166. WHO Monograph Series, No. 56, Annex 7.

APPENDIX E

American Thoracic Society Dyspnea Scale

Grade	Degree	
0	None	Not troubled with breathlessness except with strenuous exercise.
1	Slight	Troubled by shortness of breath when hurrying on the level or walking up a slight hill.
2	Moderate	Walks slower than people of the same age on the level because of breathlessness or has to stop for breath when walking at own pace on the level.
3	Severe	Stops for breath after walking about 100 yards or after a few minutes on the level.
4	Very severe	Too breathless to leave the house or breathless when dressing or undressing.

From Brooks SM (chairman). Task group on surveillance for respiratory hazards in the occupational setting. Surveillance for respiratory hazards. ATS News 1982; 8: 12–16, with permission.

APPENDIX F

Medical Research Council's Questionnaire on Respiratory Symptoms

Breathlessness

If the subject is disabled from walking by any condition other than heart or lung disease, omit Question 8 and enter 1 here   _____

8a. Are you troubled by shortness of breath when hurrying on level ground or walking up a slight hill?   _____

If Yes
8b. Do you get short of breath with other people of your own age on level ground?   _____

If Yes
8c. Do you have to stop for breath when walking at your own pace on level ground?   _____

From Medical Research Council's Committee on Environmental and Occupational Health. Questionnaire on Respiratory Symptoms. London, Medical Research Council, 1986; 2, with permission.

APPENDIX G

Visual Analogue Scale

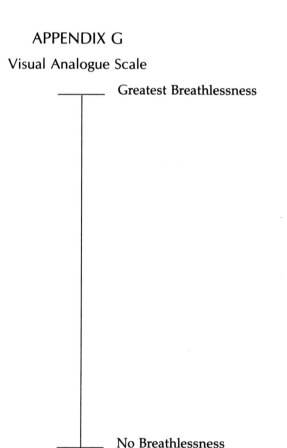

Greatest Breathlessness

No Breathlessness

From Mahler DA. Dyspnea: diagnosis and management. Clin Chest Med 1987; 8: 215–230, with permission.

APPENDIX H

Oxygen-Cost Diagram

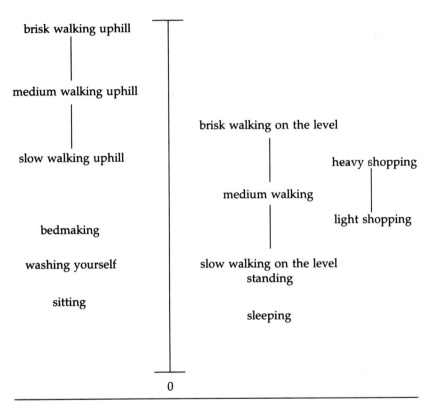

From McGavin CR, Artvinli M, Naoe H, et al. Dyspnea, disability, and distance walked: comparison of estimates of exercise performance in respiratory disease. Br Med J 1978; 2:241–243, with permission.

APPENDIX I

Baseline Dyspnea Index

Functional Impairment

_____ **Grade 4:** **No Impairment.** Able to carry out usual activities and occupation without shortness of breath.

_____ **Grade 3:** **Slight Impairment.** Distinct impairment in at least one activity but no activities completely abandoned. Reduction, in activity at work **or** in usual activities, that seems slight or not clearly caused by shortness of breath.

_____ **Grade 2:** **Moderate Impairment.** Patient has changed jobs **and/or** has abandoned at least one usual activity due to shortness of breath.

_____ **Grade 1:** **Severe Impairment.** Patient unable to work **or** has given up most or all usual activities due to shortness of breath.

_____ **Grade 0:** **Very Severe Impairment.** Unable to work **and** has given up most or all usual activities due to shortness of breath.

_____ **W:** **Amount Uncertain.** Patient is impaired due to shortness of breath, but amount cannot be specified. Details are not sufficient to allow impairment to be categorized.

_____ **X:** **Unknown.** Information unavailable regarding impairment

_____ **Y:** **Impaired for Reasons Other than Shortness of Breath.** For example, musculoskeletal problem or chest pain.

Usual activities refer to requirements of daily living, maintenance or upkeep of residence, yard work, gardening, shopping, etc.

Magnitude of Task

_____ **Grade 4:** **Extraordinary.** Becomes short of breath only with extraordinary activity such as carrying very heavy loads on the level, lighter loads uphill, or running. No shortness of breath with ordinary tasks.

_____ **Grade 3:** **Major.** Becomes short of breath only with such major activities as walking up a steep hill, climbing more than three flights of stairs, or carrying a moderate load on the level.

_____ **Grade 2:** **Moderate.** Becomes short of breath with moderate or average tasks such as walking up a gradual hill, climbing less than three flights of stairs, or carrying a light load on the level.

_____ **Grade 1:** **Light.** Becomes short of breath with light activities such as walking on the level, washing or standing.

_____ **Grade 0:** **No Task.** Becomes short of breath at rest, while sitting, or lying down.

_____ **W:** **Amount Uncertain.** Patient's ability to perform tasks is impaired due to shortness of breath, but amount cannot be specified. Details are not sufficient to allow impairment to be categorized.

_____ **X:** **Unknown.** Information unavailable regarding limitation of magnitude of task.

_____ **Y:** **Impaired for Reasons Other than Shortness of Breath.** For example, musculoskeletal problem or chest pain.

Magnitude of Effort

_____ **Grade 4:** **Extraordinary.** Becomes short of breath only with the greatest imaginable effort. No shortness of breath with ordinary effort.

_____ **Grade 3:** **Major.** Becomes short of breath with effort distinctly submaximal, but of major proportion. Tasks performed without pause unless the task

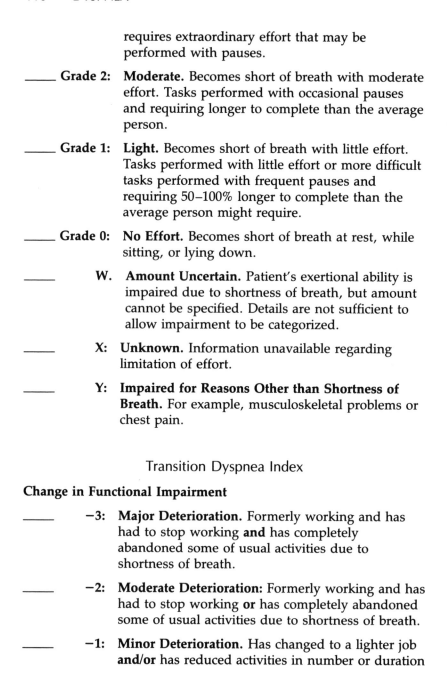

requires extraordinary effort that may be performed with pauses.

_____ **Grade 2:** **Moderate.** Becomes short of breath with moderate effort. Tasks performed with occasional pauses and requiring longer to complete than the average person.

_____ **Grade 1:** **Light.** Becomes short of breath with little effort. Tasks performed with little effort or more difficult tasks performed with frequent pauses and requiring 50–100% longer to complete than the average person might require.

_____ **Grade 0:** **No Effort.** Becomes short of breath at rest, while sitting, or lying down.

_____   **W.** **Amount Uncertain.** Patient's exertional ability is impaired due to shortness of breath, but amount cannot be specified. Details are not sufficient to allow impairment to be categorized.

_____   **X:** **Unknown.** Information unavailable regarding limitation of effort.

_____   **Y:** **Impaired for Reasons Other than Shortness of Breath.** For example, musculoskeletal problems or chest pain.

Transition Dyspnea Index

Change in Functional Impairment

_____   **−3:** **Major Deterioration.** Formerly working and has had to stop working **and** has completely abandoned some of usual activities due to shortness of breath.

_____   **−2:** **Moderate Deterioration:** Formerly working and has had to stop working **or** has completely abandoned some of usual activities due to shortness of breath.

_____   **−1:** **Minor Deterioration.** Has changed to a lighter job **and/or** has reduced activities in number or duration due to shortness of breath. Any deterioration less than preceding categories.

_____ 0: **No Change.** No change in functional status due to shortness of breath.

_____ +1: **Minor Improvement.** Able to return to work at reduced pace **or** has resumed some customary activities with more vigor than previously due to improvement in shortness of breath.

_____ +2: **Moderate Improvement.** Able to return to work at nearly usual pace **and/or** able to return to most activities with moderate restriction only.

_____ +3: **Major Improvement.** Able to return to work at former pace **and** able to return to full activities with only mild restriction due to improvement of shortness of breath.

_____ Z: **Further Impairment for Reasons Other than Shortness of Breath.** Patient has stopped working, reduced work, or has given up or reduced other activities for other reasons. For example, other medical problems, being "laid off" from work, etc.

Change in Magnitude of Task

_____ −3: **Major Deterioration.** Has deteriorated two grades or greater from baseline status.

_____ −2: **Moderate Deterioration.** Has deteriorated at least one grade but less than two grades from baseline status.

_____ −1: **Minor Deterioration.** Has deteriorated less than one grade from baseline. Patient with distinct deterioration within grade, but has not changed grades.

_____ 0: **No Change.** No change from baseline.

_____ +1: **Minor Improvement.** Has improved less than one grade from baseline. Patient with distinct improvement within grade, but has not changed grades.

_____   +2: **Moderate Improvement.** Has improved at least one grade but less than two grades from baseline.

_____   +3: **Major Improvement.** Has improved two grades or greater from baseline.

_____   Z: **Further Impairment for Reasons Other than Shortness of Breath.** Patient has reduced exertional capacity, but not related to shortness of breath. For example, musculoskeletal problem or chest pain.

Change in Magnitude of Effort

_____   −3: **Major Deterioration.** Severe decrease in effort from baseline to avoid shortness of breath. Activities now take 50–100% longer to complete than required at baseline.

_____   −2: **Moderate Deterioration.** Some decrease in effort to avoid shortness of breath, although not as great as preceding category. There is greater pausing with some activities.

_____   −1: **Minor Deterioration.** Does not require more pauses to avoid shortness of breath, but does things with distinctly less effort than previously to avoid breathlessness.

_____   0: **No Change.** No change in effort to avoid shortness of breath.

_____   +1: **Minor Improvement.** Able to do things with distinctly greater effort without shortness of breath. For example, may be able to carry out tasks somewhat more rapidly than previously.

_____   +2: **Moderate Improvement.** Able to do things with fewer pauses and distinctly greater effort without shortness of breath. Improvement is greater than preceding category, but not of major proportion.

_____   +3: **Major Improvement.** Able to do things with much
              greater effort than previously with few, if any,
              pauses. For example, activities may be performed
              50–100% more rapidly than at baseline.

_____   Z: **Further Impairment for Reasons Other than
              Shortness of Breath.** Patient has reduced exertional
              capacity, but not related to shortness of breath.
              For example, musculoskeletal problem or chest
              pain.

From Mahler DA, Weinberg DH, Wells CK, et al. The measurement of dyspnea:
Contents, interobserver agreement, and physiologic correlates of two new clinical
indexes. Chest 1984; 85:751–758, with permission.

APPENDIX J

The Modified Baseline Dyspnea Index

I. Criteria for Grade Assignment: Functional Impairment at Work

Grade 4: **No Impairment.** The patient is able to carry out usual job-related activities without shortness of breath. To be classified as grade 4, the patient should:

(a) *not* have changed jobs or job activities as a result of shortness of breath.

(b) *not*, for reasons of shortness of breath, have decreased the amount of hours/week (s)he works, or curtailed any job-related activities because they were too strenuous, either by eliminating certain tasks in the same job or by changing jobs to a less physically demanding one.

Grade 3: **Slight Impairment.** The patient recognizes that shortness of breath has caused him/her to alter job activities.

Although no job responsibilities have been completely abandoned as a result of shortness of breath, at least one job-related task is done more slowly due to shortness of breath.

Grade 2: **Moderate Impairment.** The patient has:

(a) maintained the same job and same hours/week as before the onset of dyspnea but, because of shortness of breath, has abandoned completely at least one of the tasks (s)he had done as part of that job, or

(b) changed jobs to a less strenuous position, because shortness of breath interfered with job activities, or

(c) maintained his/her previous job (e.g., the job (s)he had before dyspnea began), but decreased the number of hours/week worked at that job.

Categories (b) and (c) are not mutually exclusive, as when the patient decreases the amount of hours on one job but adds a second, less strenuous job for financial reasons. This situation is also coded as grade 2.

Grade 1: **Severe Impairment.** The patient no longer works because of shortness of breath. This category would include:

(a) Patients who have retired *early* from their job because of shortness of breath and who, despite a desire to work, have not found a realistically limited job because of shortness of breath.

(b) Patients who reached expected retirement age and stopped working and who also have dyspnea are graded according to how their shortness of breath affected their job *before* retiring. **Example:** A construction worker who left the work crew to take a desk job because of shortness of breath and who has now reached retirement age would be assigned grade 2 for "functional impairment at work" rather than grade 1.

W: **Amount Uncertain.** Patient is impaired due to shortness of breath, but amount cannot be specified because details are not sufficient.

X: **Unknown.** Information unavailable.

Y: **Impaired for Reasons Other than Shortness of Breath.** Grade Y is assigned if the patient has a main limitation due to a disability *other* than shortness of breath, e.g., chest pain, hip disease, or some other musculoskeletal impairment.

Please describe the nature of the other limiting condition(s):

Z: The patient has not had a job since before symptoms of shortness of breath began and has not since sought work.

Example: A non-breadwinner who had not intended to find a job even before shortness of breath began.

For patients who were not working when their shortness

of breath began but who have since begun to work and found shortness of breath to be a factor in determining their job, code as grade 2.

II. Criteria for Grade Assignment: Functional Impairment at Home

Grade 4:   **No Impairment.** The patient is able to carry out usual home activities without shortness of breath; there is no curtailment of the *number* or *type* of home activities, and no reduction in *pace* with which the activities are done.

Grade 3:   **Slight Impairment.** The patient recognizes that shortness of breath has caused him/her to alter the usual home activities in any of the following way(s):

(a) Although no usual activities have been completely abandoned as a result of shortness of breath, up to several (but *not all*) activities are done more slowly.

(b) Although the patient continues all his/her activities, at least one activity may be done less frequently as a result of shortness of breath.

Examples: A devoted baseball fan who, on account of shortness of breath, now goes only to an occasional game rather than his previous pattern of going to every one would be graded as having slight impairment (grade 3) in functional impairment at home.

Grade 2:   **Moderate Impairment.** Shortness of breath has caused the patient to curtail activities in at least one of the following ways:

(a) Up to several (but *not all*) activities have been *completely abandoned* because of shortness of breath, and/or

(b) Most or all usual activities are done more slowly because of shortness of breath.

Example: A patient attended the theater regularly before the onset of dyspnea but no longer attends because of his pulmonary disability. Because he still maintains his woodworking hobby at home, however, (even though he uses the tools more slowly), he should be assigned a grade 2.

Grade 1: **Severe Impairment.** Shortness of breath has caused the patient to abandon most or all of his/her usual activities.

Examples would include:

(a) The patient who is too breathless to leave the house without assistance.

(b) The patient who, as a result of shortness of breath, has come to depend on a spouse or assistant to take over the tasks of shopping, cooking, and cleaning, and who may even need help in dressing or bathing.

W: **Amount Uncertain.**

X: **Unknown.**

Y: **Impaired for Reasons Other than Shortness of Breath.** Please describe the nature of the other limiting condition(s):

III. Instructions for Assigning Composite Functional Grade

Work Functional Grade	Home Functional Grade	Composite Functional Grade
2, 3, or 4	2, 3, or 4	The lower grade in either "work" or "home" category becomes the composite grade; for identical grades in "work" and "home" categories, the composite grade is that same grade.
1 2, 3, or 4	2, 3, or 4 1	Assign composite grade as Grade 1, or severe impairment.
1	1	Assign composite grade as Grade 0, or very severe impairment. Recipients of Grade 0 will no longer be working due to shortness of breath (i.e., functional Grade 1 on work) *and* will be severely impaired in their usual home activities.

2, 3, or 4	W, X, or Y	Assign the work functional grade as the composite grade.
W, X, Y, or Z	1, 2, 3, or 4	Assign the home functional grade as the composite grade.
W, X, Y, or Z	W, X, or Y	Assign as a composite grade the two letter combination (in order with "work" grade first) of each of the individual grades; i.e., "work" grade W and "home" grade X would be composite grade WX, etc.

IV. Criteria for Grade Assignment: Magnitude of Task

Grade 4: **Extraordinary.** Becomes short of breath *only* with extraordinary activity, such as:
—carrying very heavy loads on the level
—carrying lighter loads upstairs
—running

Grade 3: **Major.** Becomes short of breath only with major activities, such as:
—walking up a steep hill
—climbing *two* flights of stairs or more
—carrying a heavy bag of groceries on the level

Grade 2: **Moderate.** Becomes short of breath with moderate or average tasks, such as:
—climbing up stairs up to two flights
—walking up a gradual hill
—walking briskly on the level
—carrying a light load on the level

Grade 1: **Light.** Becomes short of breath with light activities, such as:
—walking on the level with others of the same age
—walking to the bathroom in residence
—washing up
—dressing
—shaving

Grade 0:   No Task. Becomes short of breath with no activity, such as:
   —while sitting and/or lying down
   —while standing motionless

   W: Amount uncertain.
   X: Unknown.
   Y: Impaired for Reasons Other than Shortness of Breath.
   Please describe the nature of this other limiting condition(s):

   V. Criteria for Grade Assignment: Magnitude of Effort
For the most strenuous task the patient can perform (for at least five minutes):

Grade 4:   It is done *briskly* without pausing because of shortness of breath or even slowing down to rest.

Grade 3:   It is done *slowly* but without pausing or stopping to catch breath.

Grade 2:   It is done *slowly* and still with rare pauses (one or two) to catch breath before completing the task or quitting all together.

Grade 1:   It is done *slowly* and with many stops or pauses before the task is completed or abandoned.

Grade 0:   The patient is short of breath at rest, or while sitting, or lying down.

   W: Amount Uncertain.
   X: Unknown.
   Y: Impaired for Reasons Other than Shortness of Breath.
   Please describe the nature of this other limiting condition(s):

Note that the condition other than breathlessness that limits the patient's most strenuous condition need not be the same disability that limits the other activities described in this questionnaire. For example, the patient whose angina only occurs with strenuous activity may have little functional limitation at a sedentary job (Grade 4 for "functional impairment at work") but be limited in his/her most strenuous activity by angina (Grade Y on "magnitude of effort": chest pain).

From Stoller JK, Ferranti R, Feinstein AR. Further specifications of a new clinical index for dyspnea. Am Rev Respir Dis 1986; 134:1129–1134, with permission.

APPENDIX K

Summary of the Chronic Respiratory Disease Questionnaire:
Dyspnea Component

The questionnaire begins by eliciting five activities in which the patient experiences dyspnea during day to day activities:

1. I would like you to think of the activities that you have done during the last 2 weeks that have made you feel short of breath. These should be activities which you do frequently and which are important in your day to day life. Please list as many activities as you can that you have done during the last 2 weeks that have made you feel short of breath. (Circle the number on the answer sheet list adjacent to each activity mentioned. If an activity mentioned is not on the list, write it in, in the respondent's own words, in the space provided.)

Can you think of any other activities you have done during the last 2 weeks that have made you feel short of breath?
(Record additional items)

2. I will now read a list of activities which make some people with lung problems feel short of breath. I will pause after each item long enough for you to tell me if you have felt short of breath doing that activity during the last 2 weeks. If you haven't done the activity during the last 2 weeks, just answer "No." The activities are:
(Read items, omitting those which respondent has volunteered spontaneously. Pause after each item to give respondent a chance to indicate whether he/she has been short of breath while performing that activity during the last week. Circle the number adjacent to appropriate items on answer sheet.)

1. Being angry or upset
2. Having a bath or shower
3. Bending
4. Carrying, such as carrying groceries
5. Dressing
6. Eating
7. Going for a walk
8. Doing your housework
9. Hurrying
10. Lying flat

11. Making a bed
12. Mopping or scrubbing the floor
13. Moving furniture
14. Playing with children or grandchildren
15. Playing sports
16. Reaching over your head
17. Running, such as for a bus
18. Shopping
19. Talking
20. Vacuuming
21. Walking around your own home
22. Walking uphill
23. Walking upstairs
24. Walking with others on level ground
25. Preparing meals
26. While trying to sleep

If more than five items have been listed the interviewer then helps the subject determine the five activities which are most important in the subject's day to day life.

3. Of the items which you have listed, which is the most important to you in your day to day life? I will read through the items, and when I am finished I would like you to tell me which is the most important. (Read through all the items spontaneously volunteered and those from the list which patient mentioned.)

Which of these items is most important to you in your day to day life? (List item on response sheet.)

This process is continued until the five most important activities are determined. The interviewer then proceeds to find out how much shortness of breath the subject has experienced during the prior two weeks. Throughout the questionnaire, response options are printed on different color cards with which the subject is presented.

4. I would now like you to describe how much shortness of breath you have experienced during the last 2 weeks while doing the five most important activities you have selected.

Please indicate how much shortness of breath you have had during the last 2 weeks while (Interviewer: Insert activity list in 3) by choosing one of the following options from the card in front of you (green card):

1. Extremely short of breath
2. Very short of breath
3. Quite a bit short of breath
4. Moderate shortness of breath
5. Some shortness of breath
6. A little shortness of breath
7. Not at all short of breath

This process continues until the subject's degree of dyspnea on all five of his or her most important activities has been determined.

Information summarized from Guyatt GH, Berman LB, Townshend M, et al. A measure of quality of life for clinical trials in chronic lung disease. Thorax 1987; 42:773–778.

APPENDIX L

Borg Category Scale

0	Nothing at all
0.5	Very, very slight (just noticeable)
1	Very slight
2	Slight
3	Moderate
4	Somewhat severe
5	Severe
6	
7	Very severe
8	
9	Very, very severe (almost maximal)
10	Maximal

Modified from Borg GAV. Psychophysical bases of perceived exertion. Med Sci Sports Exerc 1982; 14:377–381.

References

1. Stevens SS. On the theory of scales of measurement. Science 1946; 103: 677-680.
2. Feinstein AR. An additional basic science for clinical medicine: IV. The development of clinimetrics. Ann Intern Med 1983; 99:843-848.
3. Nocturnal Oxygen Therapy Trial Group. Continuous or nocturnal oxygen therapy in hypoxemic chronic obstructive lung disease. Ann Intern Med 1980; 93:391-398.
4. Emirgil C, Sobol BJ, Norman J, et al. A study of the long-term effect of therapy in chronic obstructive pulmonary disease. Am J Med 1969; 47: 367-377.
5. Burrows B, Earle RH. Course and prognosis of chronic obstructive lung disease. N Engl J Med 1969; 280:397-404.
6. Nunally JC. Psychometric Theory, 2nd Edition. New York, McGraw-Hill, 1978.
7. Kirshner B, Guyatt G. A methodological framework for assessing health indices. J Chronic Dis 1985; 38:27-36.
8. Stevens SS. Mathematics, measurement, and psychophysics. In: Stevens SS (ed). Handbook of Experimental Psychology. New York, J Wiley & Sons, Inc., 1951; 1-49.
9. Guyatt G, Walter S, Norman G. Measuring change over time: assessing the usefulness of evaluative instruments. J Chronic Dis 1987; 40:171-178.
10. Fletcher CM. The clinical diagnosis of pulmonary emphysema—an experimental study. Proc R Soc Med 1952; 45:577-584.
11. Schilling RSF, Hughes JPW, Dingwall-Fordyce I. Disagreement between observers in an epidemiological study of respiratory disease. Br Med J 1955; 1:65-68.
12. Fletcher CM, Elmes PC, Wood CH. The significance of respiratory symptoms and the diagnosis of chronic bronchitis in a working population. Br Med J 1959; 1:257-266.
13. From Rose GA, Blackburn H, Gillum RF, et al. Cardiovascular Survey Methods, 2nd Edition. Geneva, World Health Organization, 1982; 166. WHO Monograph Series, No. 56, Annex 7.
14. Brooks SM (chairman). Task group on surveillance for respiratory hazards in the occupational setting. Surveillance for respiratory hazards. ATS News 1982; 8:12-16.
15. Medical Research Council's Committee on Environmental and Occupational Health. Questionnaire on Respiratory Symptoms. London, Medical Research Council, 1986; 2.
16. Aitken RCB. Measurement of feelings using visual analogue scales. Proc R Soc Med 1969; 62:989-993.
17. Price DD, McGrath PA, Rofii A, et al. The validation of visual analogue scales as ratio scale measures for chronic and experimental pain. Pain 1983; 17:45-56.
18. Mahler DA. Dyspnea: diagnosis and management. Clin Chest Med 1987; 8:215-230.

19. Gift AG. Validation of a vertical visual analogue scale as a measure of clinical dyspnea. Rehab Nurs 1989; 14:323-325.
20. Cockcroft A, Adams L. Measurement and mechanisms of breathlessness. Bull Eur Physiopathol Respir 1986; 22:85-92.
21. McGavin CR, Artvinli M, Naoe H, et al. Dyspnea, disability, and distance walked: comparison of estimates of exercise performance in respiratory disease. Br Med J 1978; 2:241-243.
22. Mahler DA, Weinberg DH, Wells CK, et al. The measurement of dyspnea: contents, interobserver agreement, and physiologic correlates of two new clinical indexes. Chest 1984; 85:751-758.
23. Stoller JK, Ferranti R, Feinstein AR. Further specifications of a new clinical index for dyspnea. Am Rev Respir Dis 1986; 134:1129-1134.
24. Guyatt GH, Berman LB, Townshend M, et al. A measure of quality of life for clinical trials in chronic lung disease. Thorax 1987; 42:773-778.
25. Guyatt GH, Thompson PJ, Berman LB, et al. How should we measure function in patients with chronic heart and lung disease? J Chronic Dis 1985; 38:517-524.
26. Mahler DA, Wells CK. Evaluation of clinical methods for rating dyspnea. Chest 1988; 93:580-586.
27. Mahler DA, Harver A, Rosiello RA, et al. Measurement of respiratory sensation in interstitial lung disease: evaluation of clinical dyspnea ratings and magnitude scaling. Chest 1989; 96: 767-771.
28. Murciano D, Auclair MH, Pariente R, et al. A randomized, controlled trial of theophylline in patients with severe chronic obstructive pulmonary disease. N Engl J Med 1989; 320:1521-1525.
29. Harver A, Mahler DA, Daubenspeck JA. Targeted inspiratory muscle training improves respiratory muscle function and reduces dyspnea in patients with chronic obstructive pulmonary disease. Ann Intern Med 1989; 111:117-124.
30. Mahler DA, Rosiello RA, Harver A, et al. Comparison of clinical dyspnea ratings and psychophysical measurements or respiratory sensation in obstructive airway disease. Am Rev Respir Dis 1987; 135:1229-1233.
31. Cockcroft A, Adams L, Guz A. Assessment of breathlessness. Q J Med 1989; 72:669-676.
32. Woodcock AA, Gross ER, Gellert A, et al. Effects of dihydrocodeine, alcohol, and caffeine on breathlessness and exercise tolerance in patients with chronic obstructive lung disease and normal blood gases. N Engl J Med 1981; 305:1611-1616.
33. Eaton ML, MacDonald FM, Church TR, et al. Effects of theophylline on breathlessness and exercise tolerance in patients with chronic airflow obstruction. Chest 1982; 82:538-542.
34. Lane R, Cockcroft A, Adams L, et al. Arterial oxygen saturation and breathlessness in patients with chronic obstructive airways disease. Clin Sci 1987; 72:693-698.
35. Efthimiou J, Fleming J, Gomes C, et al. The effect of supplementary oral nutrition in poorly nourished patients with chronic obstructive pulmonary disease. Am Rev Respir Dis 1988; 137:1075-1082.

36. Mahler DA, Matthay RA, Snyder PE, et al. Sustained-release theophylline reduces dyspnea in nonreversible obstructive airway disease. Am Rev Respir Dis 1985; 131:22-25.
37. Guyatt GH, Townsend M, Pugsley SO, et al. Bronchodilators in chronic air-flow limitation. Am Rev Respir Dis 1987; 135:1069-1074.
38. Beau JHS, Maissiat JM. Recherches sur le mecanisme des mouvements respiratoires. Arch Gen Med 1842; 15:397-415.
39. Magendie F. Precis elementaire de physiologie. In: Flint A Jr. The Physiology of Man. New York, Appleton, 1871; 353-415.
40. Turner-Warwick M, Burrows B, Johnson A. Cryptogenic fibrosing alveolitis: clinical features and their influence on survival. Thorax 1980; 35: 171-180.
41. Mier-Jedrzejowicz A, Brophy C, Moxham J, et al. Assessment of diaphragm weakness. Am Rev Respir Dis 1988; 137:877-883.
42. Wolkove N, Dajczman E, Colacone A, et al. The relationship between pulmonary function and dyspnea in obstructive lung disease. Chest 1989; 96:1247-1251.
43. Jones NL, Jones G, Edwards RHT. Exercise tolerance in chronic airway obstruction. Am Rev Respir Dis 1971; 103:477-491.
44. Mahler DA, Harver A. Prediction of peak oxygen consumption in obstructive airway disease. Med Sci Sports Exercise 1988; 20:574-578.
45. Means JH. Dyspnea. Medicine 1924; 3:309-416.
46. Sturgis CC, Peabody FW, Hall FC, et al. Clinical studies on the respiration. VIII. The relation of dyspnea to the maximum minute volume of the pulmonary ventilation. Arch Intern Med 1931; 29:236-244.
47. Hugh-Jones P, Lambert AV. A simple standard exercise test and its use for measuring exertion dyspnoea. Br Med J 1952; 1:65-71.
48. Gaensler EA, Wright GW. Evaluation of respiratory impairment. Arch Environ Health 1966; 12:146-189.
49. Warring FC Jr. Ventilatory function. Am Rev Tuberc 1945; 51: 432-454.
50. Jones NL. Clinical Exercise Testing, 3rd Edition. Philadelphia, W.B. Saunders Company, 1988; 74-122.
51. Borg G. Perceived exertion as an indicator of somatic stress. Scand J Rehab Med 1970; 2:92-98.
52. Borg GAV. Psychophysical bases of perceived exertion. Med Sci Sports Exercise 1982; 14:377-381.
53. Killian KJ, Campbell EJM. Dyspnea and exercise. Ann Rev Physiol 1983; 45:465-479.
54. Killian KJ, Jones NL. The use of exercise testing and other methods in the investigation of dyspnea. Clin Chest Med 1984; 5:99-108.
55. Killian KJ. The objective measurement of breathlessness. Chest 1985; 88(suppl):84S-90S.
56. El-Manshawi A, Killian KJ, Summers E, et al. Breathlessness during exercise with and without resistive loading. J Appl Physiol 1986; 61:896-905.
57. LeBlanc P, Bowie DM, Summers E, et al. Breathlessness and exercise in patients with cardiorespiratory disease. Am Rev Respir Dis 1986; 133: 21-25.

58. Wilson RC, Jones PW. A comparison of the visual analogue scale and modified Borg scale for the measurement of dyspnea during exercise. Clin Sci 1989; 76:277-282.
59. Silverman M, Barry J, Hellerstein H, et al. Variability of the perceived sense of effort in breathing during exercise in patients with chronic obstructive pulmonary disease. Am Rev Respir Dis 1988; 137:206-209.
60. Stark RD, Gambles SA, Lewis JA. Methods to assess breathlessness in healthy subjects: a critical evaluation and application to analyze the acute effects of diazepam and promethazine on breathlessness induced by exercise or by exposure to raised levels of carbon dioxide. Clin Sci 1981; 61:429-439.
61. Stark RD, Gambles SA, Chatterjee SS. An exercise test to assess clinical dyspnea; estimation of reproducibility and sensitivity. Br J Dis Chest 1982; 76:269-278.
62. Adams L, Chronos N, Lane R, et al. The measurement of breathlessness induced in normals: validity of two scaling techniques. Clin Sci 1985; 69:7-16.
63. Adams L, Lane R, Shea SA, et al. Breathlessness during different forms of ventilatory stimulation: a study of mechanisms in normal subjects and respiratory patients. Clin Sci 1985; 69:663-672.
64. Lane R, Adams L, Guz A. Is low-level respiratory resistive loading during exercise perceived as breathlessness? Clin Sci 1987; 73:627-634.
65. O'Neill PA, Stark RD, Allen SC, et al. The relationship between breathlessness and ventilation during steady-state exercise. Bull Eur Physiopathol Respir 1986; 22:247-250.
66. Mahler DA, Faryniarz K, Olmstead EM, et al. Breathlessness during exercise in asthma. Am Rev Respir Dis 1989; 139(suppl): A626.
67. O'Neill PA, Stretton TB, Stark RD, et al. The effect of indomethacin on breathlessness in patients with diffuse parenchymal disease of the lung. Br J Dis Chest 1986; 80:72-79.
68. Light RW, Muro JR, Sato RI, et al. Effects of oral morphine on breathlessness and exercise tolerance in patients with chronic obstructive pulmonary disease. Am Rev Respir Dis 1989; 139:126-133.
69. Swinburn CR, Wakefield JM, Jones PW. Relationship between ventilation and breathlessness during exercise in chronic obstructive airways disease is not altered by prevention of hypoxaemia. Clin Sci 1984; 67:515-519.
70. Davidson AC, Leach R, George RJD, et al. Supplemental oxygen and exercise ability in chronic obstructive airways disease. Thorax 1988; 43: 965-971.
71. Mahler DA, Faryniarz K, Lentine T, et al. Measurement of breathlessness during exercise in asthmatics: predictor variables, reliability, and responsiveness. (Submitted for publication).
72. Harver A, Mahler DA, Daubenspeck JA, et al. Multivariate support for three distinct approaches to the assessment of respiratory sensation in patients with obstructive lung disease. In: Proceedings of the VII International Symposium on Respiratory Psychophysiology. von Euler C, Katz-Salamon M (eds). New York, Stockton Press, 1988; 103-112.

Chapter 4

Acute Dyspnea

Donald A. Mahler

I. Introduction

This chapter describes the etiologies, diagnostic tests, and relevant therapies for the problem of acute dyspnea. The onset of breathlessness may occur with explosive rapidity and lead to a feeling of impending doom. Consequently, the individual patient frequently goes to an Emergency Department (ED) for evaluation and treatment.

In one community hospital, 2.7% of all ED visits over a 5 week period were due to a primary complaint of breathlessness.[1] Fifty-two percent of these patients were admitted to the hospital, which comprised 16% of non-surgical admissions.[1] This figure is similar to previous reports of 21% to 25% from hospitals in England.[2,3] Overall,

From *Dyspnea*, edited by Donald A. Mahler, M.D., © 1990, Futura Publishing Company, Inc., Mount Kisco, NY.

these percentages reflect the seriousness of the complaint of acute breathlessness and its impact on hospital resources. Congestive heart failure, asthma, and COPD accounted for 26%, 25%, and 15% of the diagnoses, respectively.[1]

II. Etiologies of Acute Dyspnea

Clinical and radiographic findings associated with the various etiologies for acute dyspnea are listed in Table 1.

Table 1. Characteristics of Various Etiologies for Acute Dyspnea

Disorder	Clinical Findings	Chest Radiograph
Airway obstruction: laryngospasm	stridor; possible allergic reaction; shock;	
aspirated foreign body	history of choking; gurgling respirations;	
bronchoconstriction	history of airway disease; wheezing	hyperinflation with flattened diaphragms
Hyperventilation syndrome	recent emotional upset; neurotic personality	normal
Chest trauma: fractured ribs	tenderness on chest palpation;	disruption of rib shadows;
pneumothorax	unilateral hyperresonance; diminished or absent breath sounds	air in pleural space with collapse of lung; shift or mediastinum if tension
Pneumonia	fever; purulent sputum	parenchymal infiltrate
Pulmonary edema: cardiogenic	frothy sputum; cyanosis; crackles	cardiomegaly; pleural effusions
noncardiogenic	frothy sputum; cyanosis; crackles	normal heart size
Pulmonary embolism	pleuritic chest pain; predisposing risk factors	may be normal; atelectasis; oligemia; pleural effusion; consolidation
Pulmonary hemorrhage	hemoptysis	focal or diffuse alveolar infiltrates; may clear within 24–48 hours
Spontaneous pneumothorax	unilateral hyperresonance; diminished or absent breath sounds	air in pleural space with collapse of lung; shift of mediastinum if tension

A. Airway Obstruction

1. Upper Airway

In adults, acute development of upper airway obstruction generally is due to aspiration of a foreign body, blunt trauma, malignancies, retropharyngeal abscess, epiglottitis, and anaphylaxis.[4] If the lesion is extra-thoracic (above the sternal notch), inspiratory stridor may be a prominent physical finding when auscultating the neck.[5] Therapy depends on the specific etiology.

In adults, aspiration of a foreign body usually occurs during a meal.[6] "Cafe coronary" occurs when a bolus of food, frequently a piece of meat, becomes lodged in the hypopharynx and upper larynx and causes partial or complete airway obstruction as well as aphonia. This situation can be mistaken for a myocardial infarction. The typical victim is middle-aged or elderly, wears dentures, and has been drinking alcohol, which diminishes protective upper respiratory reflexes. The patient may be unable to breathe or talk and exemplifies a panic-type facial expression. The usual response is for the individual to clutch one or both hands over the front of his/her neck and to struggle in an attempt to breathe. This is considered the "universal distress signal."[7]

The Heimlich maneuver, also described as "subdiaphragmatic abdominal thrusts," is recommended for relieving foreign body airway obstruction.[7,8] This maneuver elevates the diaphragm and can force air from the lungs in sufficient quantity to create an artificial cough to expel an obstructing foreign body. The rescuer's hands should never be placed on the xiphoid process of the sternum or on the lower margins of the rib cage.[7] Rather, they should be above the umbilicus but below the xiphoid process. If the victim is conscious and either standing or seated, the rescuer should stand behind the victim, wrap his/her arms around the victim's waist, and grasp one fist with the other hand. The rescuer should then press the fist into the victim's abdomen (or lower one half of the sternum) with a quick upward thrust. Each new thrust should be a separate and distinct movement.[7]

If the victim is unconscious and lying down, the rescuer should kneel astride the victim's thighs and place the heel of one hand against the victim's abdomen. The second hand should be placed directly on top of the other hand. The rescuer should then press into the abdomen with a quick upward thrust. It may be necessary to repeat the thrust 6 to 10 times to clear the airway.[7]

If a foreign body can be seen in the mouth, it should be removed with the fingers. The finger sweep should only be performed on an unconscious individual.[7]

Non-penetrating trauma to the upper airway generally consists of sports injuries in young adult men and blunt trauma from motor vehicle accidents.[4] Hoarseness may be the major symptom, while swelling and crepitus are important physical findings. Depending on the severity of injury, some patients may require endotracheal intubation, cricothyrotomy, or even tracheostomy.

Upper airway obstruction can occur within minutes of an anaphylactic reaction. Angioneuritic edema can develop in the tongue, lips, and laryngeal area due to release of mediators from an allergic response. Identifiable antigens include hymenoptera (bee) stings, ingestion of shellfish, and drug reactions, although many other antigens are possible. Management involves establishment of an airway and administration of epinephrine.

2. Bronchoconstriction

Acute bronchoconstriction may develop in any individual with hyperreactive airways, especially asthma and chronic obstructive pulmonary disease (COPD). Sudden bronchospasm can develop as a result of a respiratory infection, exposure to allergens, inhalation of fumes, dusts, and other airway irritants, environmental factors such as cold ambient air, ingestion of various foods/liquids, and even emotional stress. However, a respiratory tract infection, particularly viral, is probably the most frequent precipitating factor in acute asthma.[9] Airway obstruction is due not only to bronchial smooth muscle constriction, but also to mucosal edema and excessive mucous production. Predominant symptoms include breathlessness, wheezing, and coughing. Severe airflow obstruction may contribute to orthopnea and even inability to sleep at night.

A majority of patients who develop acute bronchoconstriction will have a history of asthma or COPD. Only a minority of individuals who experience an acute attack will be unfamiliar with the problem or cause. In obtaining a pertinent history, the physician should focus on four points:[10] (1) Can a precipitating factor be identified? Recent history of a respiratory tract infection would strongly suggest the diagnosis; (2) What medications has the individual been taking? Aspirin or beta-adrenergic antagonists may contribute to bronchoconstriction. Recent use of bronchodilators is essential in planning initial therapy;

(3) Does the patient have any known allergies? (4) Are there other concurrent medical conditions? For example, a history of heart disease may raise the consideration of "cardiac asthma" due to congestive heart failure.

Physical examination should be brief and focus on vital signs and the cardiopulmonary systems. A rapid respiratory rate ($\geq$ 30 breaths/min) and heart rate ($\geq$ 120 beats/min) indicate severe physiological impairment. Blood pressure should be examined for evidence of pulsus paradoxus. Kelsen and colleagues[11] have suggested that a pulsus paradoxus of greater than 20 mmHg usually means that asthma is severe enough to require hospitalization. Actually, an increased difference in systolic blood pressure with the phases of respiration is not paradoxical, but rather an exaggerated response to a pathophysiological process. The upper airway should be closely examined in order to exclude an obstruction due to tumor, goiter, or foreign body masquerading as an asthma attack.[12] Physical findings of the chest may vary from nearly absent breath sounds (poor air movement) to diffuse, bilateral wheezing over the chest on inspiration and especially with expiration.[5]

Ideally, peak expiratory flow (PF) or spirometry should be measured to confirm the diagnosis and to determine the severity of physiological impairment.[13] In general, the forced expiratory volume in one second (FEV_1) needs to fall below 25% of the age-related predicted value before an increase in arterial carbon dioxide tension ($PaCO_2$) occurs.[13,14] Thus, the percent of predicted value for PF and/or FEV_1 along with pulse oximetry for measuring oxygen saturation (SaO_2) are useful parameters for non-invasive assessment of gas exchange.

A chest radiograph is not indicated for all patients with acute bronchospasm. However, if the history and/or examination is suggestive of either a pneumothorax or pneumonia, then chest films are appropriate.

Several comparative studies of various bronchodilators have been performed to evaluate optimal therapy of acute asthma in the ED.[15-22] Current data indicate that inhaled beta-adrenergic therapy given 20 minutes apart for 3 doses provides comparable improvement in lung function as achieved with 3 doses of parental epinephrine.[16] The inhalational route of delivery is effective even in patients with severe airflow obstruction.[16,19]

Recommended initial therapy for acute asthma treated in the office or in the ED is 0.5 mL (2.5 mg) of albuterol in 2.5 mL of normal saline via nebulizer every 20 minutes for 3 doses. Lung function (PF or FEV_1) should be remeasured 60 minutes after the first treatment or sooner if there is marked clinical improvement. Fanta et al.[18] have demonstrated that patients with persistent severe obstruction (FEV_1 ≤ 40% of predicted) after the first hour of intensive therapy will manifest little further improvement over the ensuing three hours of emergency room care despite continued aggressive bronchodilator therapy (Figure 1). Thus, if PF or FEV_1 is less than 40% of predicted

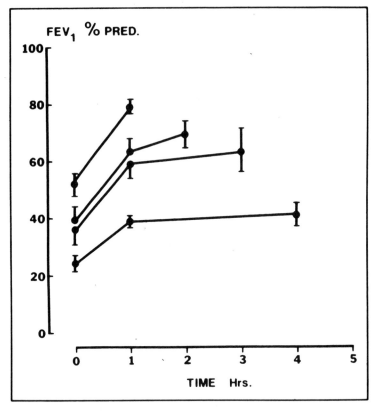

Figure 1. *Response of forced expiratory volume in one second (FEV_1) to intensive bronchodilator therapy in asthmatic patients with FEV_1 less than 40% of predicted after the first hour of treatment in the Emergency Department. Therapy included nebulized beta-adrenergic agonist (isoproterenol) every 20 minutes for three doses and then hourly at 60 minutes as well as subcutaneous terbutaline given at 60 minutes. (Adapted from Fanta CH, Rossing TH, McFadden ER Jr. Emergency room treatment of asthma: relationships among therapeutic combinations, severity of obstruction, and time course of response. Am J Med 1982; 72:416-422, with permission.)*

after three doses of nebulized albuterol, the patient should be considered for hospital admission. Several studies have shown that if the PF or FEV_1 is less than 55% to 60% of predicted at the time of discharge from the ED, it is likely that a relapse or respiratory difficulties will occur which may require repeat treatment in the ED and subsequent admission to the hospital.[13,23–25] On the other hand, if the PF or FEV_1 is greater than 60% of predicted after treatment, there is a resonable expectation that the patient can be successfully discharged home.[13,23–25] These guidelines for emergency evaluation and treatment of acute asthma are summarized in Table 2.

Table 2. Guidelines for Emergency Evaluation and Treatment of Acute Bronchoconstriction

1. Measure FEV_1 or PF initially.

2. If FEV_1 or PF is less than 25% of predicted, measure arterial blood gases. Expect that $PaCO_2 \geq 40$ mmHg.

3. Treat with inhaled beta-2 adrenergic agonist—0.5 ml (2.5 mg) of albuterol in 2.5 ml of normal saline—via nebulizer every 20 minutes for three doses.

4. Repeat measurement of FEV_1 or PF 60 minutes later or sooner if marked clinical improvement (see Figure 1).

5. If FEV_1 or PF

    < 40% of predicted:

  a. Consider hospitalization;
  b. Give intravenous corticosteroids (methylprednisolone 40 to 125 mg every 6 hrs);
  c. Give intravenous aminophylline (or theophylline) if patient is going to be hospitalized (loading dose: 4–5 mg/kg over 30 min if no recent theophylline therapy; otherwise, give maintenance dose of 0.5 to 0.9 mg/kg/hr).

    40% to 60% of predicted:

  a. Individual judgement required for decision to hospitalize or discharge.

    > 60% of predicted:

  a. Anticipate discharge home;
  b. Consider brief course of oral corticosteroids (7 to 14 days) if patient is discharged in addition to beta-2 adrenergic agonist metered-dose inhaler and oral sustained-release theophylline.

B. Chest Trauma

Penetrating and non-penetrating trauma to the chest can cause a myriad of injuries which range from minimal impairment to life threatening. This discussion will focus on injuries which predominantly cause breathlessness as the primary symptom. The two major conditions are pneumothorax and pulmonary contusion.

1. Pneumothorax

Air in the pleural space may arise from the tracheobronchial tree or from an injury to the chest wall, such as with fractured ribs or penetrating trauma. Rupture of the tracheobronchial tree typically involves the trachea or proximal main bronchi within 2 to 3 cm of the main carina and may be associated with fracture of the first three ribs.[26] The diagnostic triad of tracheobronchial rupture is pneumothorax, hemoptysis, and subcutaneous/mediastinal emphysema.[27] Single or multiple fractures of the ribs can rupture the parietal pleura and lead to a pneumothorax. Localized chest wall pain is usually a prominent associated symptom. At times, positive pressure can develop within the pleural space causing a tension pneumothorax and resultant shift of the central structures to the opposite side. Hypotension and shock can develop. Immediate release of the tension is essential using a needle with syringe or chest tube.

2. Pulmonary Contusion

Pulmonary contusion is the most frequent radiographic finding in patients with severe blunt chest injury.[28] The radiographic patterns include patchy densities presumably representing blood distributed along the distal bronchial-pulmonary sheaths and a homogenous alveolar infiltrate consisting of blood/fluid in alveoli. Hemoptysis may be present. Typically, a pulmonary contusion appears within the first few hours after chest trauma and resolves over several days. Aspiration pneumonitis should be considered in the differential diagnosis, although the radiographic picture generally involves the lower lung fields and may be diffuse. Treatment involves supportive care, including supplemental oxygen and/or mechanical ventilation, depending on the severity of impairment in gas exchange.

C. Hyperventilation Syndrome

The hyperventilation syndrome is a clinical term usually reserved for hyperventilation and respiratory alkalosis due to emotional factors and/or anxiety.[29] It has also been termed "psychogenic dyspnea." The incidence of this problem has been estimated to be from 6% to 11%.[30-32] Most studies indicate that the hyperventilation syndrome is two to four times more common in women than in men and occurs predominantly in the third to fourth decades of life.[29] Breathlessness occurs in 50%–90% of patients with hyperventilation syndrome and is rarely related to exertion.[29] Burns and Howell[33] reported that sudden onset with rapid increase in dyspnea was characteristic of those with "disproportionate" breathlessness. Fluctuating and recurrent episodes of breathlessness are common.[33] Hyperventilation leads to a decrease in $PaCO_2$ and respiratory alkalosis which causes vasoconstriction of cerebral arteries. This decrease in cerebral blood flow may be responsible for the dizziness, faintness, visual disturbances, and impaired psychomotor behavior that are commonly described during hyperventilation.[34] Chest pain can be a prominent symptom, although typically there is no relationship between exertion and onset of the chest pain. Numbness and tingling of the fingers, toes, and perioral areas may be associated complaints. Anxiety is the major psychogenic cause for the hyperventilation syndrome. In patients with "disproportionate" breathlessness, there was a strikingly high incidence of obsessional personality.[33]

The diagnosis depends on a high index of suspicion by the physician. Clues to the presence of the hyperventilation syndrome are listed in Table 3. The presence of a normal chest radiograph, a decrease in $PaCO_2$, and a normal alveolar-arterial oxygen difference strongly support the diagnosis. Currently, hyperventilation syndrome, or psychogenic dyspnea, remains a diagnosis of exclusion.

Compernolle et al.[35] have suggested that the diagnosis can be confirmed by voluntary hyperventilation (hyperventilation provocation test). The patient is instructed to breathe deeply and rapidly in an attempt to reproduce symptoms; generally, two to three minutes of vigorous hyperventilation are sufficient.[36] Once symptoms are produced, the acute episode can be terminated by having the patient rebreathe into a bag.

Although hypocapnia is characteristic of the hyperventilation syndrome, the use of arterial blood gases for the diagnosis can be

Table 3. Clues to the Presence of the Hyperventilation Syndrome
1. Female, 20 to 40 years of age.
2. Many vague and unrelated minor complaints.
3. Concern about a life-threatening illness.
4. Has visited numerous physicians.
5. Feels "nervous," and "nervousness" is common in the family.
6. Marital and sexual problems.
7. Breathlessness and chest pain are not related to exertion.
8. Occasional sighing or yawning.

Adapted from Brashear RE. Hyperventilation syndrome. Lung 1983; 161:257–273.

confusing. The finding of a decreased $PaCO_2$ and an elevated pH may simply reflect acute hyperventilation in response to the anticipated discomfort and apprehension associated with sampling of arterial blood.

Although reassurance and/or rebreathing into a bag can resolve the acute symptoms of the hyperventilation syndrome, appropriate treatment should focus on anxiety as the etiology. Treatment strategies include psychotherapy, psychotropic drugs, beta-adrenergic blocking drugs, and behavior therapy.[29]

Diaphragmatic flutter may be initially misdiagnosed as intractable hyperventilation attacks.[37] Kondo et al.[37] have described three patients who demonstrated a fast respiratory rhythm (230–250 breaths/min) superimposed on a slow rhythm (15–30 breaths/min). The fast rhythm maintained arterial blood gases at normal or hypocapnic levels. The dual rhythms were diagnosed by recording volume or air flow during an attack. Diaphragmatic flutter includes clonic contractions of the diaphragm and other respiratory muscles and occurs only when patients are awake.[38] Intravenous diphenylhydantoin and intramuscular haloperidol can suppress the abnormal respiratory patterns.[37]

D. Pneumonia

Fever, purulent sputum, and a parenchymal infiltrate on chest radiographs are the usual findings in bacterial pneumonia. Dyspnea is a frequently associated complaint even in previously healthy individuals. Empiric antibiotic therapy may be appropriate based on the clinical suspicion of a pathogen, the age of the patient, and the severity of illness. In immunocompromised hosts, identification of a specific organism is essential. If an adequate sputum sample cannot be obtained, then transtracheal aspiration or fiberoptic bronchoscopy should be considered to obtain lower respiratory tract secretions for smears and cultures in selected patients.

E. Pulmonary Edema

Pulmonary edema can be classified according to the permeability of the vascular endothelium. Normal permeability pulmonary edema can be due to increased intravascular hydrostatic pressure (Table 4), decreased oncotic gradient (rarely), and decreased lymphatic clearance (unusual as primary cause).[39] A recently described cause of pulmonary edema related to increased hydrostatic pressure is the use of beta-adrenergic agonists to arrest uterine contractions in pregnant women.[40] Symptoms include acute dyspnea (76%), chest pain (24%), and cough (17%). The onset of symptoms occurs before delivery in 70% of cases, but also may develop within 12 hours after delivery.[40]

Increased permeability pulmonary edema may result from a va-

Table 4. Conditions that Increase Intravascular Hydrostatic Pressure

1. Increased left ventricular end-diastolic pressure
   a. cardiac disease (coronary artery, valvular, and cardiomyopathy)
   b. intravenous fluid overload
   c. high output states (thyrotoxicosis, arteriovenous fistula)
   d. systemic hypertension
   e. tocolytic therapy (drugs used to inhibit uterine contractions)
2. Increased left atrial pressure
   a. mitral valve disease
   b. left atrial myxoma
3. Increased pulmonary venous pressure
   a. pulmonary veno-occlusive disease
   b. fibrosing mediastinitis
4. Neurogenic edema
   a. head trauma
   b. seizures
   c. cerebrovascular accident
5. High-altitude pulmonary edema

Table 5. Major Causes of Increased Permeability
1. Aspiration
2. Drug overdose
3. Inhalation of toxic chemicals
4. Pancreatitis
5. Sepsis
6. Shock
7. Trauma

riety of insults to the endothelial or epithelial surfaces (Table 5). Dyspnea is the most frequent symptom of these conditions and may be associated with orthopnea, paroxysmal nocturnal dyspnea, and chest pain. Interstitial edema may stimulate juxtacapillary receptors as a neuro-medicated afferent signal to contribute to breathlessness.[41]

The diagnosis depends on the clinical information along with chest radiographic findings. In some instances the measurement of pulmonary artery occlusion (wedge) pressure (PAOP) may be necessary to distinguish normal permeability (high PAOP) from increased permeability (low or normal PAOP) edema.

Treatment depends on the cause of pulmonary edema.[39] When increased hydrostatic pressure leads to transudation of fluid, supplemental oxygen and diuretic therapy generally are beneficial. Supportive care is indicated for neurogenic causes of pulmonary edema. Supplemental oxygen and rapid descent are important for high altitude pulmonary edema. Increased permeability pulmonary edema frequently leads to the adult respiratory distress syndrome (ARDS); supplemental oxygen, intubation, and mechanical ventilation frequently are required.

F. Pulmonary Embolism

Most patients with pulmonary emboli have recognizable predisposing conditions (Table 6). However, there are no clinical findings specific for the diagnosis. Chest pain appears to be the most common complaint and is frequently, but not always, pleuritic.[42] Dyspnea is nearly a universal symptom (84%) and appears to be unrelated to the extent of pulmonary emboli.[42] It is possible that receptors in the pulmonary circulation and/or right heart may contribute to the sensation of breathlessness in pulmonary embolism.[43,44]

The diagnosis depends on ventilation-perfusion mismatching on

Table 6. Risk Factors for Thomboembolism
1. Stasis of venous circulation
a. immobilization
b. venous disease
c. congestive heart failure
d. obesity
2. Trauma
a. burns
b. surgery
c. childbirth
d. fractures
3. Estrogens
4. Malignancy
5. Advanced age
6. Previous history of thromboembolism
7. Hypercoagulable state

lung scan and/or evidence of thrombophlebitis by studies of the lower extremities. Pulmonary arteriography may be necessary in selected cases. Acute therapy includes intravenous heparin or thrombolysis (if massive pulmonary embolism with severe cardiovascular compromise, hypotension, and/or shock), followed by heparin therapy.

G. Pulmonary Hemorrhage

Acute pulmonary hemorrhage is an unusual but potentially life-threatening cause of the sudden onset of dyspnea. If the bleeding is diffuse, respiratory failure and even death due to asphyxiation can ensue. The presence of hemoptysis is an important symptom that usually suggests the possibility of pulmonary hemorrhage. Frequent causes of pulmonary hemorrhage include vasculitis, especially Goodpasture's syndrome and Wegener's granulomatosis, bronchogenic carcinoma, bronchial adenoma, bronchiectasis, lung abscess, tuberculosis, and mycetoma. In some instances, the patient may be able to localize the bleeding site to one side of the chest. Fiberoptic bronchoscopy is generally performed to investigate the etiology. An open lung biopsy may be necessary to establish a diagnosis of vasculitis.

H. Spontaneous Pneumothorax

Spontaneous pneumothorax occurs when a subpleural bleb or an alveolus ruptures into the pleural space. Approximately 75% of cases occur with sedentary activity, whereas about 20% are associated with strenuous activities and the remaining 5% occur with coughing, sneezing, and wheezing.[45] In over 1600 episodes of pneumothorax compiled by Killen and Gobbel,[46] 98% were symptomatic. Chest pain and dyspnea are the two most common symptoms of spontaneous pneumothorax. The pain usually is localized or unilateral; it may be constant or may have a pleuritic component. Dyspnea is the second most common symptom, and its severity depends on the extent of the pneumothorax as well as the presence of underlying lung function. Spontaneous pneumothorax may be primary or secondary to one of several respiratory diseases (Table 7). For many patients, the sudden onset of both chest pain and dyspnea prompt evaluation in the Emergency Department. In a small percentage of patients, a tension pneumothorax can develop; the increased pressure within the pleural space can shift the mediastinum and compress central blood vessels, compromising venous return and leading to hypotension and shock.

If the pneumothorax is small in size and cardiorespiratory function is well maintained, no specific therapy may be indicated. However, most episodes of spontaneous pneumothorax respond to evacuation of air by placement of a chest tube into the pleural space. A tension pneumothorax requires urgent release of pressure within the pleural space by inserting a needle connected to a syringe or a chest tube.

Table 7. Causes of Secondary Spontaneous Pneumothorax

1. Bacterial pneumonia, especially Staphylococcus aureus which can cause abscess formation and pneumatoceles.
2. Catamenial endometriosis.
3. Chronic obstructive pulmonary disease.
4. Cystic fibrosis.
5. Interstitial lung disease, especially the late stages of sarcoidosis and eosinophilic granuloma.
6. Malignancy, especially sarcoma and lymphoma.
7. Marfan's syndrome.
8. Status asthmaticus due to increased intra-alveolar pressure.
9. Tuberculosis.

III. Summary

Acute dyspnea may represent the major symptom of a life-threatening illness or injury. Therefore, prompt evaluation and therapy are critical. The physician should ask four "key" questions to assess the various causes of acute breathlessness.[47] These are the following:

1. *Are you short of breath at rest?* Breathlessness at rest suggests severe physiological impairment.

2. *Do you have any chest pain? If so, where is it located?* Localized or unilateral chest pain may suggest a spontaneous pneumothorax, pulmonary embolism, or possible chest trauma. Substernal chest pain or heaviness may indicate a myocardial infarction as a cause for pulmonary edema. Patients with hyperventilation syndrome may note discomfort over the left breast area.

3. *What were you doing before and at the onset of breathlessness?* The patient is usually aware of an injury, fall, or accident that may have caused upper airway or chest trauma. Most occurances of spontaneous pneumothorax occur with sedentary activity, although roughly 20% develop with exertion. In pulmonary embolism, there may be a history of prolonged travel, recent surgery, immobilization of a lower extremity, etc. Ingestion of specific foods or a recent bee sting suggests possible laryngeal edema.

4. *Do you have any major medical or surgical conditions?* A history of asthma raises the possibility of acute bronchospasm. Chronic respiratory diseases, especially cystic fibrosis and COPD, are important causes of a secondary spontaneous pneumothorax. A past history of ischemic heart disease may predispose to pulmonary edema. Use of tocolytic therapy (drugs that inhibit uterine contractions) in a pregnant woman can be associated with pulmonary edema.

Diagnostic tests depend on the differential diagnosis generated by the combined results from the history and physical examination. Guidelines for specific therapy are provided in major medical and surgical textbooks.

References

1. Fedullo AJ, Swinburne AJ, McGuire-Dunn C. Complaints of breathlessness in the emergency department. N Y State J Med 1986; 86:4-6.
2. Pearson SB, Pearson EM, Mitchell JR. The diagnosis and management of

patients admitted to hospital with breathlessness. Postgrad Med J 1981; 57:419-424.

3. Mustchin CP, Tiwari I. Diagnosing the breathless patient (letter). Lancet 1982; i:907-908.

4. Jacobson S. Upper airway obstruction. Emerg Med Clin North Am 1989; 7:205-217.

5. Baughman RP, Loudon RG. Stridor: differentiation from asthma or upper airway noise. Am Rev Respir Dis 1989; 139:1407-1409.

6. Eller WC, Haugen RK. Food aspiration—restaurant rescue. N Engl J Med 1973; 289:81-82.

7. American Heart Association. Healthcare Provider's Manual for Basic Life Support. 1988; 35-59.

8. Heimlich HJ. A life-saving maneuver to prevent food-choking. JAMA 1975; 234:398-401.

9. Hudgel DW, Langston L Jr, Selner JC, et al. Viral and bacterial infections in adults with chronic asthma. Am Rev Respir Dis 1979; 120:393-397.

10. Scoggins CH. Acute asthma and status asthmaticus. In: Sahn SA (ed). Pulmonary Emergencies. New York, Churchill Livingston, 1982; 127-148.

11. Kelsen SG, Kelsen DP, Fleegler BF, et al. Emergency room assessment and treatment of patients with acute asthma: adequacy of the conventional approach. Am J Med 1978; 64:622-628.

12. Shim C, Corro P, Park SS, et al. Pulmonary function studies in patients with upper airway obstruction. Am Rev Respir Dis 1972; 106:233-238.

13. Nowak RM, Tomlanovich MC, Sarkar DD, et al. Arterial blood gases and pulmonary function testing in acute bronchial asthma: predicting patient outcomes. JAMA 1983; 249:2043-2046.

14. McFadden ER Jr, Lyons HA. Arterial blood gas tensions in asthma. N Engl J Med 1968; 278:1027-1032.

15. Josephson GW, MacKenzie EJ, Lietman PS, et al. Emergency treatment of asthma: a comparison of two treatment regimens. JAMA 1979; 242:639-643.

16. Rossing TH, Fanta CH, Goldstein DH, et al. Emergency therapy of asthma: comparison of acute effects of parental and inhaled sympathomimetics and infused aminophylline. Am Rev Respir Dis 1980; 122:365-371.

17. Rossing TH, Fanta CH, McFadden ER Jr. A controlled trial of the use of single versus combined-drug therapy in the treatment of acute episodes of asthma. Am Rev Respir Dis 1981; 123:190-194.

18. Fanta CH, Rossing TH, McFadden ER Jr. Emergency room treatment of asthma: relationships among therapeutic combinations, severity of obstruction, and time course of response. Am J Med 1982; 72:416-422.

19. Fanta CH, Rossing TH, McFadden ER Jr. Treatment of acute asthma: is combination therapy with sympathomimetics and methylxanthines indicated? Am J Med 1986; 80:5-10.

20. Siegel D, Sheppard D, Gelb A, et al. Aminophylline increases the toxicity but not the efficacy if an inhaled beta-adrenergic agonist in the treatment of acute exacerbations of asthma. Am Rev Respir Dis 1985; 132:283-286.

21. Bryant DH. Nebulized ipratropium bromide in the treatment of acute asthma. Chest 1985; 88:24-29.
22. Karpel JP, Appel D, Briedbart D, et al. A comparison of atropine sulfate and metaproterenol sulfate in the emergency treatment of asthma. Am Rev Respir Dis 1986; 133:727-729.
23. Banner AS, Shah RS, Addington WW. Rapid prediction of need for hospitalization in acute asthma. JAMA 1976; 235:1337-1338.
24. Nowak RM, Gordon KR, Wroblewski DA, et al. Spirometric evaluation of acute bronchial asthma. J Am Coll Emerg Phys 1979; 8: 9-12.
25. Nowak RM, Pensler MI, Sarkar DD, et al. Comparison of peak expiratory flow and FEV_1 admission criteria for acute bronchial asthma. Ann Emerg Med 1982; 11:64-69.
26. Kirsh MM, Orringer MB, Behrendt DM, et al. Management of tracheobronchial disruption secondary to nonpenetrating trauma. Ann Thorac Surg 1976; 22:93-101.
27. Chesterman JT, Satsangi PN. Rupture of the trachea and bronchi by closed injury. Thorax 1966; 21:21-27.
28. Hopeman AR. Chest trauma. In: Sahn SA (ed). Pulmonary Emergencies. New York, Churchill Livingston, 1982; 342-344.
29. Brashear RE. Hyperventilation syndrome. Lung 1983; 161:257-273.
30. Rice RL. Symptom patterns of the hyperventilation syndrome. Am J Med 1950; 8:691-700.
31. Singer EP. The hyperventilation syndrome in clinical medicine. N Y State J Med 1958; 58:1494-1500.
32. Yu PN, Yim JB, Stanfield CA. Hyperventilation syndrome. Arch Intern Med 1959; 103:902-913.
33. Burns BH, Howell JBL. Disproportionately severe breathlessness in chronic bronchitis. Q J Med 1969; 38:277-294.
34. Lum LC. Hyperventilation: the tip and the iceberg. J Psychosom Res 1975; 19:375-383.
35. Compernolle T, Hoogduin K, Joele L. Diagnosis and treatment of the hyperventilation syndrome. Psychosomatics 1979; 20:612-625.
36. Stead EA, Warren JV. The role of hyperventilation in the production, diagnosis, and treatment of certain anxiety symptoms. Am J Med Sci 1943; 206:183-190.
37. Kondo T, Tamaya S, Ohta Y, et al. Dual-respiratory rhythms: a key to diagnosis of diaphragmatic flutter in patients with HVS. Chest 1989; 96: 106-109.
38. Phyllips JR, Eldredge FL. Respiratory myoclonus (Leeuwenhoeck disease). N Engl J Med 1973; 289:1390-1395.
39. Fishman AP. Pulmonary edema. In: Fishman AP (ed). Pulmonary Diseases and Disorders, 2nd Edition. New York, McGraw-Hill, 1988; 919-952.
40. Pisani RJ, Rosenow EC III. Pulmonary edema associated with tocolytic therapy. Ann Intern Med 1989; 110:714-718.
41. Coleridge HM, Coleridge JCG. Reflexes evoked from tracheobronchial tree and lungs. In: Cherniack NS, Widdicombe JG (eds). Handbook of

Physiology, Section 3: The Respiratory System. Bethesda, American Physiological Society, 1986; 395-407.
42. Bell WR, Simon TL, DeMets DL. The clinical features of submassive and massive pulmonary emboli. Am J Med 1977; 62:355-360.
43. Jones PW, Huszczuk A, Wasserman K. Cardiac output as a controller of ventilation through changes in right ventricular load. J Appl Physiol 1982; 53:218-224.
44. Ledsome JR. The reflex role of pulmonary arterial baroreceptors. Am Rev Respir Dis 1977; 115:245-250.
45. Sahn S. Pneumothorax. In: Sahn SA (ed). Pulmonary Emergencies. New York, Churchill Livingston, 1982; 239-273.
46. Killen DA, Gobbel WG Jr. Spontaneous Pneumothorax. Boston, Little Brown & Co, 1968; 160-163.
47. Mahler DA. Dyspnea: diagnosis and management. Clin Chest Med 1987; 8:215-230.

Chapter 5

Positional Dyspnea

Donald A. Mahler

I. Introduction

Positional effects on dyspnea probably are more common than recognized or appreciated. Certainly any patient who complains of breathlessness should be asked whether postural changes affect shortness of breath. On the other hand, medical literature deals predominantly with physiological changes associated with different body positions. Usually, it is assumed that predictable changes in breathlessness follow alterations in physiological function and/or gas exchange. However, positional changes in dyspnea may be distinct from changes in lung mechanics and oxygenation.

From *Dyspnea*, edited by Donald A. Mahler, M.D., © 1990, Futura Publishing Company, Inc., Mount Kisco, NY.

145

In this chapter, the effect of body position on respiratory function will be described. Thereafter, the problems of positional dyspnea (trepopnea, orthopnea, and platypnea) will be explained relative to physiological changes or dysfunction. Although these descriptions may suggest a physiological explanation for the development or increase in dyspnea in a specific position, such relationships are plausible, albeit speculative. Finally, the physiology of the prone position is considered.

II. Effect of Body Position on Respiratory Function

Vertical pleural pressure gradients, which influence regional expansion of the lungs and gas distribution, exist in the chests of normal individuals.[1-4] At lung volumes above functional residual capacity (FRC), regional ventilation is greatest in the dependent lung zones because of the pressure-volume relationship of the lung.[2,4,5] Regional blood flow is determined mainly by gravitational forces. It is greatest in the dependent lung zones due to hydrostatic pressure differences within the pulmonary blood vessels (Figure 1).[2,3] As a result, regional ventilation($\dot{V}$)-perfusion($\dot{Q}$) relationships vary according to the vertical location or zone in the lung.

In healthy individuals, a change in position from seated to supine appears to have a variable effect on gas exchange.[6-9] Alterations in oxygenation with a change in posture would result from the interaction of three factors: (1) an increase in cardiac output in the supine position[10]; (2) increased uniformity of regional $\dot{V}/\dot{Q}$ relationships when supine[2]; and (3) the lung volume at which airway closure occurred.[11] Craig et al.[12] reported that there was marked intersubject variation in gas exchange in different positions based on the relationship of "closing volume" to breathing level (FRC plus tidal volume). These collective results demonstrate that arterial oxygen pressure (PaO$_2$) and the alveolar-arterial oxygen difference [(A − a) DO$_2$] are variably affected by posture in healthy subjects.

When a normal person is in a lateral decubitus position, ventilation and blood flow have the same relationship to the vertical height of the lung as when the individual is upright. The dependent lung is affected not only by gravity, but also by the hydrostatic pressure of the abdominal contents which elevates the dependent portion of the diaphragm and by the weight of the mediastinal structures.[2] The

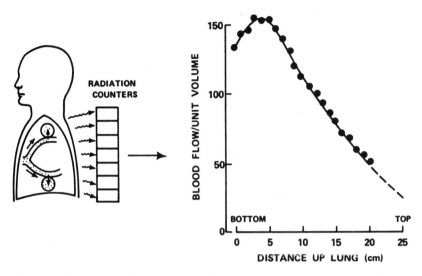

Figure 1: *Distribution of blood flow in the upright human lung using radioactive xenon. Note that blood flow is greatest in the dependent portion of the lung. (From West JB. Respiratory Physiology—The Essentials, 3rd Edition. Baltimore, Williams & Wilkins Co, 1985; 31-48, with permission.)*

resultant effects on the dependent lung are a smaller lung volume (Figure 2) but greater ventilation than the non-dependent lung (Figure 3).[5] The gravitational pressure gradient in the pulmonary vessels operates to cause greater blood flow to the dependent lung.[3] The consequent changes in ventilation and blood flow are relatively matched so that oxygenation is nearly identical in supine, right lateral, and left lateral positions in normal subjects.[13]

Despite the recognized effects of gravity and body position on cardiopulmonary function, postural changes in symptoms have not been well understood by clinicians and may thereby be neglected. Specific cardiorespiratory disorders may cause positional dyspnea (Table 1). For example, in unilateral pneumonia or unilateral pleural effusion, dyspnea may develop in one lateral position but not in the other (trepopnea). In congestive heart failure, chronic obstructive pulmonary disease (COPD), or bilateral diaphragm paralysis, lying supine may compromise respiration and contribute to breathlessness (orthopnea). Finally, in certain types of right-to-left shunts, dyspnea may be induced in the upright position and relieved by recumbency (platypnea).

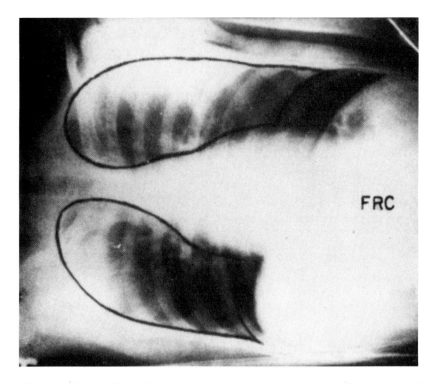

Figure 2: *Chest radiograph in the right lateral decubitus position at functional residual capacity (FRC). For comparison, the lung fields are outlined as observed in the upright position. (From Kaneko K, Milic-Emili J, Dolovich MB, et al. Regional distribution of ventilation and perfusion as a function of body position. J Appl Physiol 1966; 21:767-777, with permission.)*

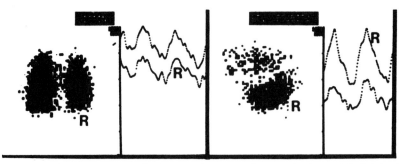

Figure 3: *A krypton-81m ventilation scan in a normal person in the upright (sitting) and right lateral decubitus position. Normally, ventilation is increased in the dependent lung. Breath-by-breath wave forms are next to the scans. (From Shim C, Chun KJ, Williams MH Jr, et al. Positional effects on distribution of ventilation in chronic obstructive pulmonary disease. Ann Intern Med 1986; 105:346-350, with permission.)*

Table 1. Various Diseases Causing Positional Dyspnea

1. Trepopnea–dyspnea in one lateral position but not in the other
   a. Unilateral lung disease
   b. Unilateral pleural effusion
   c. Unilateral obstruction of the airway
   d. Chronic obstructive pulmonary disease

2. Orthopnea–dyspnea in the recumbent position
   a. Left ventricular failure
   b Obstructive airway disease
   c. Respiratory muscle weakness/paralysis

3. Platypnea–dyspnea in the upright position and relieved by recumbency
   a. Intracardiac shunts
   b. Vascular lung shunts
      Congenital
      Acquired
   c. Parenchymal lung shunts

III. Trepopnea

Trepopnea is dyspnea in one lateral position but not in the other position. The lateral position may affect gas exchange and the development of dyspnea when a unilateral disease process exists.

Remolina et al.[14] have observed that PaO_2 was lower when the involved or "sick" lung was in the dependent position as opposed to when the uninvolved or "good" lung was dependent. Furthermore, these investigators demonstrated that the positional hypoxemia reversed upon resolution of the unilateral disease.[14] Although hypoxemia normally can influence regional blood flow distribution, gravitational forces are not affected in a major way by hypoxemia in the lateral decubitus position; blood flow is not directed up to the "good" lung when it is non-dependent.[15]

The presumed mechanism for the altered gas exchange involves positional changes in the matching of ventilation to perfusion.[14,16] When the diseased lung is dependent, gravitational forces cause enhanced blood flow, whereas regional ventilation cannot increase appropriately due to the disease itself (pneumonia, atelectasis, hemorrhage, pleural effusion, etc.). Increased $\dot{V}/\dot{Q}$ mismatching could then lead to positional hypoxemia and trepopnea. Falke et al.[17] have demonstrated that positive end-expiratory pressure (PEEP) improved oxygenation in a patient with unilateral pulmonary infiltrates only when the "good" lung was dependent. Presumably, PEEP led to regional changes in lung volume and/or blood flow and resulted in improved gas exchange.

Gillespie and Rehder[18] used the multiple inert gas elimination technique to investigate the mechanisms for the postural changes in gas exchange in patients with unilateral lung disease. Four patients with respiratory failure who required mechanical ventilation were studied. Each patient demonstrated a unilateral interstitial pattern on chest radiograph. When the "good" lung was in the dependent position, PaO_2 increased (range, 12 to 57 mmHg) in all four patients, whereas there was no change in arterial carbon dioxide pressure ($PaCO_2$). The major cause for improved oxygenation was a decrease in right-to-left shunting in two patients and enhanced $\dot{V}/\dot{Q}$ matching in the other two patients. These results emphasize the variability of mechanisms which can influence gas exchange in different body positions.

Occasionally, dyspnea may develop when the "good" lung is dependent. Mahler et al.[19] demonstrated that a patient with a left upper lobe carcinoma developed tachypnea and oxygen desaturation when lying on his right side. Fiberoptic bronchoscopy revealed a mass in the distal left main stem bronchus at the site of the left upper lobe stump (previous left upper lobe lobectomy). When the patient turned onto his right side, further narrowing of the left main stem bronchus was observed. Thus, mechanical obstruction of the left main stem bronchus decreased ventilation and presumably led to hypoxemia based on low ventilation-perfusion matching in the left lower lobe. In this specific individual, "up with the good lung" was more appropriate for his condition.

Various investigators have reported positional hypoxemia in patients with unilateral pleural effusions.[20-23] Pleural fluid decreases lung volume and causes the regional pressure in the pleural space to be less negative. These effects diminish ventilation to the lung on the same side as the effusion. However, perfusion to the lung on the involved side also may be affected. In patients with unilateral pleural effusions, $PaCO_2$ values are similar between the two lateral positions suggesting that alveolar ventilation is not measurably affected by the change in positions.[22] Sonnenblick et al.[20] concluded that the decline of PaO_2 when the involved side was dependent was attributable to mismatching of ventilation and perfusion. They performed a perfusion lung scan in a patient with a large pleural effusion and found almost no perfusion to the ipsilateral lung with the "bad" side dependent.[20] Polverino et al.[23] demonstrated better ventilation and perfusion in three patients with unilateral pleural effusions when the "good" lung was dependent as opposed to when the "sick" lung was dependent. Chang et al.[22] reported that the postural effect on gas exchange was highly correlated with measures of FEV_1 ($r = 0.74$; p < 0.001) and FVC ($r = 0.63$; p < 0.001) obtained in the erect position.

IV. Orthopnea

Orthopnea is dyspnea in the recumbent position. This symptom arises from alterations of gravitational forces when the recumbent position is assumed. In left heart failure, orthopnea develops because of redistribution of fluid from the lower extremities into the chest. The increase in central blood volume augments pulmonary capillary hydrostatic pressure and may lead to formation of interstitial edema. Juxtacapillary receptors presumably play a role for increasing afferent signals via the vagus nerve.[24,25] In severe left heart failure, the patient may not be able to lie down, but rather must remain in an upright position even when sleeping.

In severe obstructive airway disease, elevation of the hemidiaphragms and consequent reduction in FRC can further compromise diaphragm function. Despite an increase in length of the costal fibers of the diaphragm, changes in gravitational forces in the supine position require increased pleural pressure to overcome the increased hydrostatic pressure in the abdominal cavity. As a result, dyspnea may ensue. When the patient assumes an upright position, the effect of gravity increases FRC and enhances diaphragm function.

Minh et al.[26] compared supine and upright PaO_2 in 16 patients with COPD. In 8 patients in whom PaO_2 decreased in the supine position, $\dot{V}/\dot{Q}$ decreased significantly whereas venous admixture increased; in the other 8 patients, PaO_2 increased with recumbency.

Ries and colleagues[27] have examined the effect of posture on arterial oxygenation in 117 COPD patients. Compared to the supine position, there was a variable change in standing PaO_2 which increased (> 3 mmHg) in 28 patients, remained unchanged (±3 mmHg) in 57 patients, and decreased (< 3 mmHg) in 32 patients. Although substantial postural changes in PaO_2 were observed in many patients, the alterations were not predictable based on physiological parameters. Thus, it appears that changes in PaO_2 based on body position are quite variable in patients with COPD.

In addition, neuromuscular diseases can cause weakness and paralysis of the diaphragm and other respiratory muscles that accentuate positional alterations in respiratory mechanics. Orthopnea can be an early symptom of diaphragmatic weakness. In fact, patients with the lowest values for transdiaphragmatic pressure (Pdi) had the greatest degree of orthopnea[28] (Figure 4). Patients with complete paralysis of the diaphragm demonstrated paradoxical breathing (inward movement of the abdomen during inspiration) when supine.[28] Mier-Jedrzejowicz et al.[28] found that orthopnea and abdominal paradox were always present when the sniff Pdi was less than 30 cmH_2O. The authors suggest that 30 cmH_2O is the approximate pressure to overcome the hydrostatic pressure of the abdominal contents when supine.[28]

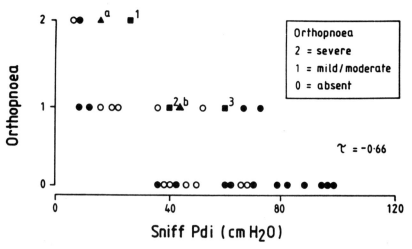

Figure 4: *Association between grade of orthopnea and transdiaphragmatic pressure during maximal sniffs (sniff Pdi) in 30 male (solid circles) and female (open circles) patients with diaphragm weakness. (From Mier-Jedrzejowicz A, Brophy C, Moxham J, et al. Assessment of diaphragm weakness. Am Rev Respir Dis 1988; 137:877-883, with permission.)*

V. Platypnea (with Orthodeoxia)

Platypnea is defined as dyspnea induced in the upright position and relieved by recumbency.[29] Usually, orthodeoxia (arterial deoxygenation in the upright position and improved with recumbency) has been observed in association with platypnea.[29] The complaint of breathlessness accentuated by sitting or standing (as opposed to lying supine) should not be interpreted as a functional disability, but rather should direct the physician to investigate a variety of possible conditions. The distinctive complex of findings has been recognized in patients with various types of shunts.[30]

A. Intracardiac Shunts

Atrial septal defects (ASD), both congenital and acquired, can cause right-to-left shunting in the upright position. This phenomenon has more recently been reported when pulmonary thromboembolism or pneumonectomy leads to a pressure-induced increase in right-to-left flow across a patent foramen ovale.[31-36] At least two different mechanisms may contribute to shunting and desaturation.[37] One possibility is that a change in the pressure gradient between right and left atria produces a right-to-left shunt or augments the magnitude of an existing shunt. This may be due to increased impedance of the pulmonary circulation relative to the systemic circulation or from an alteration in the relative positions of the two atria. Subsequently, Selzer and Lewis[36] postulated that "streaming" of blood from the inferior vena cava across the septal defect to the left atrium might occur in the absence of a pressure gradient. Franco et al.[32] performed cardiac catheterization in a patient with platypnea and orthodeoxia after a right pneumonectomy. In this patient, there was no pressure gradient observed from the right to the left atrium in either supine or upright positions. Seward et al.[35] speculated that the upright position allowed enhanced "streaming" of blood from the inferior vena cava into the left atrium (Figure 5). A second consideration is that cardiac output decreases in the presence of the existing level of oxygen consumption; this leads to desaturation of mixed venous blood with no change in the shunt fraction[37]

The diagnosis can be made non-invasively by performing tilt-table contrast two-dimensional echocardiography.[35,38] This technique

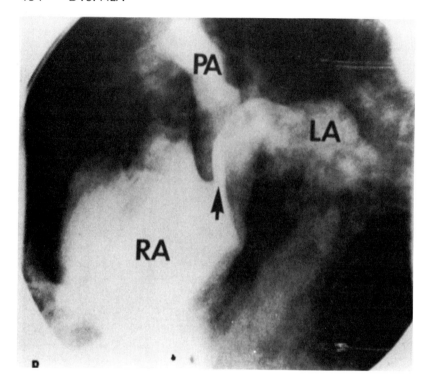

Figure 5: *Inferior vena caval angiogram in a patient with platypnea-orthodeoxia. Contrast material is shunted from the right atrium (RA) to the left atrium (LA) across the atrial septum (arrow). (From Seward JB, Hayes DL, Smith HC, et al. Platypnea-orthodeoxia: clinical profile, diagnostic workup, management, and report of seven cases. Mayo Clin Proc 1984; 59:221-231, with permission.)*

provides visualization and localization of a right-to-left shunt of less than 4% (Figure 6).[35] In most instances this procedure obviates the need for cardiac catheterization in the upright position.[35] Certainly, a high degree of clinical suspicion is critical to establish the diagnosis along with an appreciation of the association of pneumonectomy (right or left), platypnea, and orthodeoxia. The demonstration of a right-to-left intracardiac shunt is important because it is amenable to surgical correction.

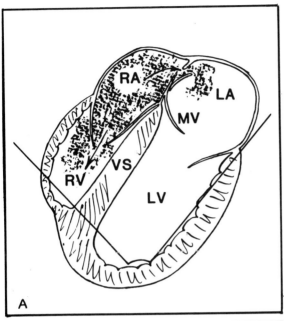

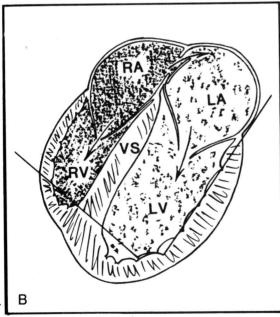

Figure 6: *Diagrams of two-dimensional contrast echocardiograms in the upright position in a patient with platypnea-orthodeoxia. Contrast material appears first in the right atrium (RA). Then, contrast normally enters the right ventricle (RV). In diagram A, contrast also crosses the atrial septum into the left atrium (LA). Subsequently, contrast enters the left ventricle (LV) as observed in diagram B. (From Seward JB, Hayes DL, Smith HC, et al. Platypnea-orthodeoxia: clinical profile, diagnostic workup, management, and report of seven cases. Mayo Clin Proc 1984; 59:221-231, with permission.)*

B. Vascular Lung Shunts

1. Congenital

Pulmonary arteriovenous malformations (PAVM) represent congenital malformations that include the spectrum of pulmonary arteriovenous connections extending from a single aneurysmal lesion to multiple microscopic communications too small to be visualized radiographically.[39,40] PAVM are variably associated (36% to 57%) with Osler-Weber-Rendu disease.[41–43] Although a majority of PAVM are congenital, the condition frequently is not recognized until the second decade of life.[44] In two series, the mean age of presentation was 39 years and 41 years.[42,43]

Shumacker and Waldhausen[44] have suggested that PAVM enlarge progressively with age in response to increased blood flow. The vessel wall may eventually necrose, which increases the magnitude of the communication. Most PAVM occur in the lower lobes of the lung.[41–43] The most common abnormality is a single circumscribed peripheral lesion connected by blood vessels to the hilus of the lung.[39] However, multiple PAVM also are common. The radiographic size of the lesion(s) appears to be related to a higher incidence of symptoms and physical findings.

Dyspnea, especially in the upright position and with exertion, develops, in part, with positional changes in blood flow through the PAVM. Pulmonary blood flow is greatest in the most dependent portions of the lung.[3,4] In the supine position, enhanced flow is directed to the dependent lung zones of the upper and lower lobes. However, in the upright position, blood flow is particularly increased to the lower lobes where PAVM are most common. Consequently, blood is shunted through PAVM more in the upright than the supine position, and platypnea with orthodeoxia results.

Associated physical findings include pulmonary vascular bruits, mucocutaneous telangiectasias, polycythemia, clubbing, and cyanosis. As part of the initial investigation of hypoxemia, measurement of shunt is recommended by obtaining arterial blood gases with the patient breathing room air and 100% oxygen in the supine and upright positions. Contrast echocardiography is useful to document the presence and site of right-to-left shunting. Normally, peripheral injection of dye generates detectable echoes that are filtered on passage through the pulmonary vasculature. In right-to-left shunts, echoes occur in the left atrium; this technique confirms the presence of shunting, but not the specific etiology. As a result, pulmonary arteriography is the "gold standard" for establishing a diagnosis of PAVM.[39]

Although the natural history of PAVM is not completely known, available clinical data suggest that treatment should be considered in all cases.[35,39] Therapeutic options include surgical resection and embolization with either a coil device or a balloon.[39,41-43,45-47] Embolotherapy is the treatment of choice for suitable patients in institutions where facilities and expertise exist.[39,47]

2. Acquired

Although rare, acquired PAVM have been reported after chest surgery, trauma, actinomycosis, cirrhosis, and metastatic carcinoma.[48] Of these etiologies, liver cirrhosis has been the most commonly recognized in association with hypoxemia, cyanosis, and clubbing.[49-53] Dilated pulmonary vascular channels and/or arteriovenous communications (lung spider nevi) have been demonstrated on pulmonary angiography and at postmortem examination. Shunting of blood does not occur only through acquired PAVM, but also by pulmonary venous blood flowing through non-ventilated alveoli and/or by dilated capillary and precapillary beds in which diffused oxygen ineffectively reaches hemoglobin.[53-55] Edell and colleagues[56] used the multiple inert gas elimination technique to demonstrate that both $\dot{V}/\dot{Q}$ mismatching and right-to-left shunting contributed to hypoxemia in patients with chronic liver disease and orthodeoxia.

Between 15% to 45% of cirrhotic patients have one or more of the following abnormalities: hypoxemia, clubbing, and hyperventilation.[57] Although a spectrum of pulmonary vascular disorders may exist in chronic liver disease, intrapulmonary shunting is probably the most important mechanism of *severe* hypoxemia. Radiographic findings may demonstrate bibasilar interstitial infiltrates, which correspond to angiographic evidence of "spongy" pulmonary vessels, and nodular shadows consistent with arteriovenous communications. Up to 20% of patients with cirrhosis may have a reduction in single-breath diffusing capacity due to shunting.[48,58]

Platypnea and orthodeoxia have been reported in up to 5% of

cirrhosis patients.[53,55,59] Because the intravascular shunts predominate in the the lung bases, redistribution of blood to the lung bases in the upright position may enhance right-to-left shunting as described for PAVM. Intrapulmonary vascular shunts may occur in the absence of portal hypertension. The diagnosis may be established by measurement of shunt in the supine and upright positions; demonstration of nodular shadows on chest radiography, especially in the lower lung zones; contrast echocardiography; and quantitative radionuclide scanning. Pulmonary arteriography generally is not necessary in the appropriate clinical setting, especially when a right-to-left, non-cardiac shunt has been demonstrated.

3. Parenchymal Lung Disease

Platypnea and orthodeoxia have been described in patients with severe COPD,[60,61] interstitial fibrosis,[62] adult respiratory distress syndrome (ARDS),[63] and autonomic failure.[64] Parenchymal lung shunts due to dilated arteriovenous vascular channels may be present in select cases.[61,62,64] Multiple small vessels acting as shunts may not be evident by the usual diagnostic tests, including pulmonary arteriography. Demonstration of a physiological shunt by measurement of PaO_2 on room air and 100% oxygen may be the only method for documenting a shunt.

In addition, $\dot{V}/\dot{Q}$ mismatching may be another mechanism for platypnea-orthodeoxia.[60,63,64]

VI. The Prone Position

Neither the development nor the relief of dyspnea in the prone position has been a prominent clinical problem. However, alterations in gas exchange can occur in patients with diffuse lung injury when positioned prone.

Computed tomography (CT) scans of lung morphology in patients with ARDS have shown that bilateral posterobasal infiltrates are quite common.[65-67] Accordingly, the prone position in bilateral ARDS has been compared to the lateral decubitus position in unilateral lung disease.[67] In 1974, Bryan[68] suggested that the prone position be used in mechanically ventilated patients. Subsequently, investigators have described improvement in oxygenation in patients with diffuse lung injury.[69,70]

Langer and colleagues[67] reported that 8 of 13 patients with ARDS had an improvement in PaO_2 of at least 10 mmHg after 30 minutes of being turned from the supine to the prone position. The remaining five patients showed no benefit in gas exchange and were considered "nonresponders" by the authors.[67] Albert et al.[71] studied the physiological mechanisms for improvement in arterial oxygenation with the prone position in dogs. Acute lung injury was induced by injection of oleic acid into the right atrium. Based on results in different groups of animals in a variety of positions, the prone position uniformly improved PaO_2. This occurred due to a reduction in intrapulmonary shunt and was not related to changes in FRC, regional diaphragmatic motion, cardiac output, or pulmonary vascular pressures.[71]

Presently, the prone position is not commonly used in the clinical treatment of ARDS because of the substantial logistical problems associated with providing care to sick patients in this position. However, the collective results of various studies[67-71] suggest that the prone position can markedly improve gas exchange in certain patients. Thus, in ARDS patients on mechanical ventilation when oxygenation is problematic, it is reasonable to try different body positions, e.g., lateral decubitus or prone.

VII. Summary

The symptom of positional dyspnea provides an important historical clue. However, the physician must be aware of the effect of different positions on breathlessness in order to ask appropriate questions. Usually, but not always, an alteration in gas exchange corresponds to the problems of trepopnea, orthopnea, and platypnea. The measurement of oxygen saturation by oximetry is an initial approach to evaluate positional hypoxemia. Additional testing is generally necessary in order to demonstrate the pathophysiological changes causing positional dyspnea and to establish a specific diagnosis.

References

1. Bryan AC, Bentivoglio LG, Beerel F, et al. Factors affecting regional distribution of ventilation and perfusion in the lung. J Appl Physiol 1964; 19:395-402.

2. Kaneko K, Milic-Emili J, Dolovich MB, et al. Regional distribution of ventilation and perfusion as a function of body position. J Appl Physiol 1966; 21:767-777.
3. West JB. Respiratory Physiology—The Essentials, 3rd Edition. Baltimore, Williams & Wilkins Co, 1985; 31-48.
4. Amis TC, Jones HA, Hughes JMB. Effect of posture on inter-regional distribution of pulmonary ventilation in man. Respir Physiol 1984; 56: 145-167.
5. Shim C, Chun KJ, Williams MH Jr, et al. Positional effects on distribution of ventilation in chronic obstructive pulmonary disease. Ann Intern Med 1986; 105:346-350.
6. Blair E, Hickman JB. The effect of change in body position on lung volume and intrapulmonary gas mixing in normal subjects. J Clin Invest 1955; 34:383-389.
7. Malmberg R. Pulmonary gas exchange at exercise and different body postures in man. Scand J Respir Dis 1966; 47:92-102.
8. Riley RL, Permutt S, Said S, et al. Effect of posture on pulmonary dead space in man. J Appl Physiol 1959; 14:339-344.
9. Ward RJ, Tolas AG, Benveniste RJ, et al. Effect of posture on normal arterial blood gas tensions in the aged. Geriatrics 1966; 21:139-143.
10. McGregor M, Adam W, Sekelj P. Influence of posture on cardiac output and minute ventilation during exercise. Circ Res 1961; 9:1089-1092.
11. LeBlanc P, Ruff F, Milic-Emili J. Effects of age and body position on "airway closure" in man. J Appl Physiol 1970; 28:448-451.
12. Craig DB, Wahba WM, Don HF, et al. "Closing volume" and its relationship to gas exchange in seated and supine positions. J Appl Physiol 1971; 31:717-721.
13. Zack MB, Pontoppidan H, Kazemi H. The effect of lateral positions on gas exchange in pulmonary disease. Am Rev Respir Dis 1974; 110:49-55.
14. Remolina C, Khan AU, Santiago TV, et al. Positional hypoxemia in unilateral lung disease. N Engl J Med 1981; 304:523-525.
15. Arborelius M Jr, Lundin G, Svanberg L, et al. Influence of unilateral hypoxia on blood flow through the lungs in man in lateral position. J Appl Physiol 1960; 15:595-597.
16. Fishman AF. Down with the good lung (editorial). N Engl J Med 1981; 304:537-538.
17. Falke KJ, Pontoppidan H, Kumar A, et al. Ventilation with end-expiratory pressure in acute lung disease. J Clin Invest 1972; 51:2315-2323.
18. Gillespie DJ, Rehder K. Body position and ventilation-perfusion relationships in unilateral lung disease. Chest 1987; 91:75-79.
19. Mahler DA, Snyder PE, Virgulto JA, et al. Positional dyspnea and oxygen desaturation related to carcinoma of the lung: up with the good lung. Chest 1983; 83:826-827.
20. Sonnenblick M, Melzer E, Rosin AJ. Body positional effect on gas exchange in unilateral pleural effusion. Chest 1983; 83:784-786.
21. Neagley SR, Zwillich CW. The effect of positional changes on oxygenation in patients with pleural effusions. Chest 1985; 88:714-717.

22. Chang SC, Shiao GM, Perng RP. Postural effect on gas exchange in patients with unilateral pleural effusions. Chest 1989; 96:60-63.
23. Polverino M, Santoriello C, Adiletta G, et al. Positional hypoxemia in unilateral pleural effusion. Am Rev Respir Dis 1989; 139 (suppl): A359.
24. Paintal AS. The nature and effects of sensory inputs into the respiratory centers. Fed Proc 1977; 36:2428-2432.
25. Rebuck AS, Slutsky AS. Control of breathing in diseases of the respiratory tract and lungs. In: Cherniack NS, Widdicombe JG (eds). Handbook of Physiology, Section 3: The Respiratory System. Bethesda, American Physiological Society, 1986; 771-791.
26. Minh VD, Chun D, Fairshter RD, et al. Supine change in arterial oxygenation in patients with chronic obstructive pulmonary disease. Am Rev Respir Dis 1986; 133:820-824.
27. Ries AL, Chang J, Kaplan RM. The effect of posture on arterial oxygenation in patients with chronic obstructive pulmonary disease (COPD). Am Rev Respir Dis 1989; 139 (suppl):A15.
28. Mier-Jedrzejowicz A, Brophy C, Moxham J, et al. Assessment of diaphragm weakness. Am Rev Respir Dis 1988; 137:877-883.
29. Altman M, Robin ED. Platypnea (diffuse zone/phenomenon). N Engl J Med 1969; 281:1347-1348.
30. Robin ED, Laman PD, Goris ML, et al. A shunt is (not) a shunt is (not) a shunt. Am Rev Respir Dis 1977; 115:553-557.
31. Schnabel TG Jr, Ratto O, Kirby CK, et al. Postural cyanosis and angina pectoris following pneumonectomy: relief by closure of an interatrial septum defect. J Thorac Surg 1956; 32:246-250.
32. Franco DP, Kinasewitz GT, Markham RV, et al. Postural hypoxemia in the postpneumonectomy patient. Am Rev Respir Dis 1984; 129:1021-1022.
33. LaBresh KA, Pietro DA, Coates EO, et al. Platypnea syndrome after left pneumonectomy. Chest 1981; 79:605-607.
34. Begin R. Platypnea after pneumonectomy. N Engl J Med 1975; 293:342-343.
35. Seward JB, Hayes DL, Smith HC, et al. Platypnea-orthodeoxia: clinical profile, diagnostic workup, management, and report of seven cases. Mayo Clin Proc 1984; 59:221-231.
36. Selzer A, Lewis AE. The occurence of chronic cyanosis in cases of atrial septal defect. Am J Med Sci 1949; 218:516-524.
37. Rehder K. Gravity, posture, and cardiopulmonary function. May Clin Proc 1984; 59:280-281.
38. Kronik G, Mosslacher H. Positive contrast echocardiography in patients with patent foramen ovale and normal right heart hemodynamics. Am J Cardiol 1982; 49:1806-1809.
39. Burke CM, Safai C, Nelson DP, et al. Pulmonary arteriovenous malformations: a critical update. Am Rev Respir Dis 1986; 134:334-339.
40. Stringer CJ, Stanley AL, Bates RC, et al. Pulmonary arteriovenous fistulas. Am J Surg 1955; 89:1054-1080.
41. Bosher LH Jr, Blake DA, Byrd BR. An analysis of the pathologic anatomy

of pulmonary arteriovenous aneurysms with particular reference to the applicability of local excision. Surgery 1959; 45:91-104.

42. Dines DE, Seward JB, Bernatz PE. Pulmonary arteriovenous fistula. Mayo Clin Proc 1983; 58:176-181.

43. Dines DE, Arms RA, Bernatz PE, et al. Pulmonary arteriovenous fistulas. Mayo Clin Proc 1974; 49:460-465.

44. Shumacker HB, Waldhausen JA. Pulmonary arteriovenous fistulas in children. Ann Surg 1963; 158:713-720.

45. Taylor BG, Cockerill EM, Manfredi F, et al. Therapeutic embolization of the pulmonary artery in pulmonary arteriovenous fistula. Am J Med 1978; 64:360-365.

46. Terry PB, Barth KH, Kaufman SL, et al. Balloon embolization for treatment of pulmonary arteriovenous fistulas. N Engl J Med 1980; 302:1189-1190.

47. Terry PB, White RI Jr, Barth KH, et al. Pulmonary arteriovenous malformations: physiologic observations and results of therapeutic balloon embolization. N Engl J Med 1983; 308:1197-1200.

48. Prager RL, Laws KH, Bender HW Jr. Arteriovenous fistula of the lung. Am Thorac Surg 1983; 26:231-239.

49. Golding PL, Smith M, Williams R. Multisystem involvement in chronic liver disease: studies on the incidence and pathogenesis. Am J Med 1973; 55:772-782.

50. Santiago SM Jr, Dalton JW Jr. Platypnea and hypoxemia in Laennec's cirrhosis of the liver. South Med J 1977; 70:510-512.

51. Wolfe JD, Tashkin DP, Holly FE, et al. Hypoxemia of cirrhosis: detection of abnormal small pulmonary vascular channels by a quantitative radionuclide method. Am J Med 1977; 63:746-754.

52. Berthelot P, Walker JG, Sherlock S, et al. Arterial changes in the lungs in cirrhosis of the liver—lung spider nevi. N Engl J Med 1966; 274:291-298.

53. Robin ED, Horn B, Goris ML, et al. Detection, quantification and pathophysiology of lung "spiders". Trans Assoc Am Physicians 1975; 88:202-216.

54. Davis HH, Schwartz DJ, Lefrak SS, et al. Alveolar-capillary oxygen disequilibrium in hepatic cirrhosis. Chest 1978; 73:507-511.

55. Robin ED, Laman D, Horn BR, et al. Platypnea related to orthodeoxia caused by true vascular shunts. N Engl J Med 1976; 294:941-943.

56. Edell ES, Cortese DA, Krowka MJ, et al. Severe hypoxemia and liver disease. Am Rev Respir Dis 1989; 140:1631-1635.

57. Krowka MJ, Cortese DA. Pulmonary aspects of chronic liver disease and liver transplantation. Mayo Clin Proc 1985; 60:407-418.

58. Stanley NN, Woodgate DJ. Mottled chest radiograph and gas transfer defect in chronic liver disease. Thorax 1972; 27:315-323.

59. Kennedy TC, Knudson RJ. Exercise-aggravated hypoxemia and orthodeoxia in cirrhosis. Chest 1977; 72:305-309.

60. Michel O, Sergysels R, Ham H. Platypnea induced by worsening of V_A/Q inhomogeneity in the sitting position in chronic obstructive lung disease. Chest 1988; 93:1108-1110.

61. Miller WC, Heard JG, Unger KM. Enlarged pulmonary arteriovenous vessels in COPD—another possible mechanism of hypoxemia. Chest 1984; 86:704-706.
62. Tenholder MF, Russell MD, Knight E, et al. Orthodeoxia: a new finding in interstitial fibrosis. Am Rev Respir Dis 1987; 136:170-173.
63. Khan F, Parekh A. Reversible platypnea and orthodeoxia following recovery from adult respiratory distress syndrome. Chest 1979; 75:526-528.
64. Fox JL, Brow E, Harrison JK, et al. Platypnea-orthodeoxia and progressive autonomic failure. Am Rev Respir Dis 1989; 140:1802-1804.
65. Gattinoni L, Mascheroni D, Torresin A, et al. Morphological response to positive end-expiratory pressure in acute respiratory failure. Computerized tomography study. Intensive Care Med 1986; 12:137-142.
66. Maunder RJ, Shuman WP, McHugh JW, et al. Preservation of normal lung region in the adult respiratory distress syndrome: analysis of computed tomography. JAMA 1986; 255:2463-2466.
67. Langer M, Mascheroni D, Marcolin R, et al. The prone position in ARDS patients: a clinical study. Chest 1988; 94:103-107.
68. Bryan AC. Comments of a devil's advocate. Am Rev Respir Dis 1974; 110 (suppl):143-144.
69. Douglas WW, Rehder K, Beynen FM, et al. Improved oxygenation in patients with acute respiratory failure: the prone position. Am Rev Respir Dis 1977; 115:559-566.
70. Piehl MA, Brown RS. Use of extreme position changes in acute respiratory failure. Crit Care Med 1976; 4:13-14.
71. Albert RK, Leasa D, Sanderson M, et al. The prone position improves arterial oxygenation and reduces shunt in oleic acid-induced acute lung injury. Am Rev Respir Dis 1987; 135:628-633.

Chapter 6

Chronic Dyspnea

Andrew L. Ries and Donald A. Mahler

From *Dyspnea*, edited by Donald A. Mahler, M.D., © 1990, Futura Publishing Company, Inc., Mount Kisco, NY.

I. Introduction

Dyspnea is an extremely common symptom in patients with respiratory and/or cardiac disorders. In fact, it is frequently the reason that a patient seeks medical care. For many patients, the exact onset of breathlessness is difficult to recall because, in part, the course has been slow and insidious. Quite often, the patient attributes the symptom to "getting old" or "being out of shape." Usually, the patient finally decides to see a physician because breathlessness affects or limits the ability to perform daily activities.

The experience of breathlessness is influenced not only by the magnitude of various physical tasks but also by the associated effort.[1-3] For example, sedentary individuals may not experience dyspnea until marked physiological impairment has developed. Generally, a substantial reduction in physiological capacity is required before dyspnea affects a person's day-to-day activities because of the large reserve in lung function. The individual may then reduce his/her activity level and/or degree of effort in order to minimize the experience of breathlessness. Consequently, the patient with chronic dyspnea usually becomes deconditioned as well.

Despite incomplete understanding about the exact mechanisms leading to the complex symptom of dyspnea, it usually is possible to identify a specific disease or condition as the primary cause of breathlessness. The major causes of chronic dyspnea are listed in Table 1. Respiratory and cardiac diseases represent the most frequent etiologies. The various conditions appear to contribute to the experience of breathlessness by one or more of three pathophysiological pathways:

1. Increased chemical or neurological drive to breathe.
2. Increased work of breathing.
3. Decreased neuromuscular power.

The following discussion covering the various causes of chronic dyspnea will focus on pertinent history, physical examination, and laboratory data *as they relate to the symptom of breathlessness*. No attempt will be made to describe the extensive characteristics of each disease; this information is available in major textbooks.

Table 1. Causes of Chronic Dyspnea

Respiratory
  Airway Disease
    Asthma
    Chronic obstructive pulmonary disease (chronic bronchitis and
      emphysema)
    Cystic fibrosis
    Upper airway obstruction
  Parenchymanl Lung Disease
    Interstitial lung disease
    Malignancy—primary or metastatic
  Pneumonia
  Pulmonary Vascular Disease
    Arteriovenous malformations
    Plexogenic pulmonary hypertension
    Thromboembolism
    Vasculitis
    Veno-occlusive disease
  Pleural Disease
    Effusion
    Fibrosis
    Malignancy
  Chest Wall Disease
    Deformities (e.g., scoliosis, kyphosis, ankylosing spondylitis)
    Obesity
    Ascites
    Pregnancy
  Respiratory Muscle Disease and/or Dysfunction
    Neuromuscular disorders (e.g., muscular dystrophy, amylotrophic
      lateral sclerosis, myasthenia gravis, polio)
    Malnutrition
    Thyroid disease
    Chronic primary fibromyalgia
Cardiovascular
    Elevated pulmonary venous pressure
    Decreased cardiac output
    Right-to-left shunt
Anemia
Deconditioning
Psychological factors

II. Causes of Chronic Dyspnea

A. Respiratory

1. Airway Disease

a. Asthma Asthma is characterized by reversible episodes of bronchoconstriction. Accordingly, dyspnea usually is episodic in asthma, and there may be symptom-free periods. Wheezing and/or coughing frequently accompany bronchospasm. For many untreated patients, the symptoms of asthma, including dyspnea, become worse during the night.[4] Lung function generally is lowest around 4 A.M.[5] (Figure 1), which corresponds to the greatest frequency of dyspneic episodes in untreated asthmatics[6] (Figure 2). Proposed mechanisms for nocturnal asthma are listed in Table 2.

Airway hyperreactivity characterizes the clinical and physiological status of patients with asthma. Various "triggers" initiate bronchoconstriction and the resultant development of dyspnea, chest tightness, and/or wheezing. Inhaled allergens are specific (unique to the individual) stimulators for acute (within minutes) and/or late-phase (4 to 8 hours after exposure) reactions. Non-specific "triggers" include dust, fumes, chemicals, cigarette smoke, exercise, cold air, or respiratory infections.

Some asthmatic patients are not always able to sense the presence of marked airway obstruction.[7] One possible explanation is that asthmatic individuals with mild to moderate airflow obstruction have a large respiratory reserve and may have relatively few symptoms. Also, those who experience more frequent "attacks" may have less severe ratings of breathlessness than asthmatics who have less frequent episodes of bronchospasm (temporal adaptation).[8] In addition, there can be marked variability in the accuracy of perception of spontaneous airway obstruction in individual asthmatic subjects.[9] Therefore, a peak flow meter may be particularly helpful for both the patient and the health-care provider to estimate the severity of airflow obstruction and to implement and assess treatment strategies.[10]

b. Chronic obstructive pulmonary disease (COPD) In contrast to asthma, the onset of dyspnea in patients with COPD generally is insidious, and the symptom progresses over long periods of time. Dyspnea on exertion is the most frequent complaint of COPD patients. The patient may unknowingly reduce his/her level of activities

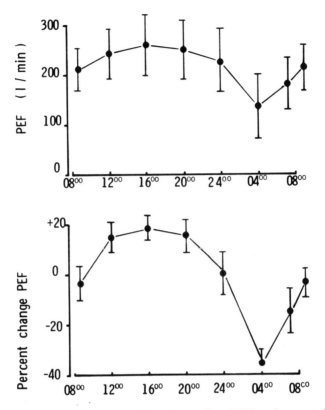

Figure 1: *Mean ± SE changes in peak expiratory flow (PEF) and percent change in PEF in upper and lower panels, respectively, over a 24-hour period in 5 patients with asthma. (From Barnes P, FitzGerald G, Brown M, et al. Nocturnal asthma and changes in circulating epinephrine, histamine, and cortisol. N Engl J Med 1980; 303:263-267, with permission.)*

in an effort to diminish the discomfort of breathlessness. This "strategy" actually complicates the disability by adding the problem of deconditioning to the exercise limitation.

Patients with COPD may also exhibit airway hyperreactivity. Exposure to cold air, exercise, and respiratory infections can lead to acute exacerbations of airflow obstruction and increased symptoms.

In addition, some patients with COPD experience disabling breathlessness when performing seemingly trivial upper extremity activities, such as combing their hair, bathing, etc.[11] Celli and col-

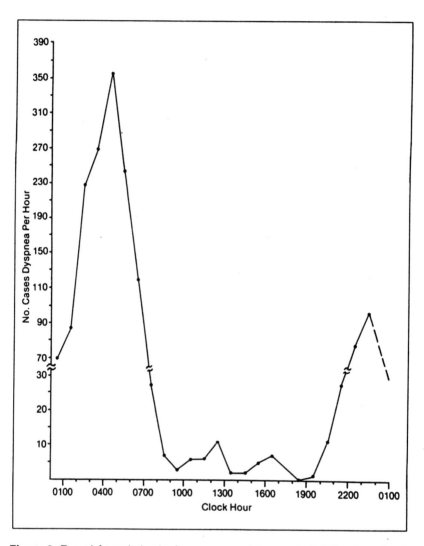

Figure 2: *Day-night variation in the occurrence of dyspnea in 3,129 untreated asth-matic patients. Most dyspneic episodes occurred between 2 A.M. and 7 A.M. (From Smolensky MH, D'Alonzo GE. Biologic rhythms and medicine. Am J Med 1988; 85(suppl):40, with permission.)*

Table 2. Proposed Mechanisms Contributing to Nocturnal Asthma

1. Late-phase reaction to allergen exposure
2. Excessive bronchial secretions
3. Impaired mucocilliary clearance
4. Airway cooling
5. Circadian rhythm
6. Gastoesophageal reflux
7. Timing and efficacy of bronchodilator medications

leagues[12] have demonstrated that during unsupported arm work, the accessory muscles of respiration help position the torso and arms. This places an increased load on the diaphragm and may thereby contribute to dyspnea.

Both an increase in the work of breathing and hyperinflation contribute to impairment in respiratory muscle function in patients with COPD. At rest, the oxygen cost of breathing is approximately 1% to 2% of total body oxygen consumption ($\dot{V}O_2$) in normal, healthy individuals, while it approaches 15% in some patients with COPD.[13,14] Although COPD is characterized by diminished expiratory airflow, the increased work of breathing is performed primarily by inspiratory muscles.[15] Hyperinflation leads to a number of problems for inspiratory muscle function[16] (Figure 3). A major effect of hyperinflation is

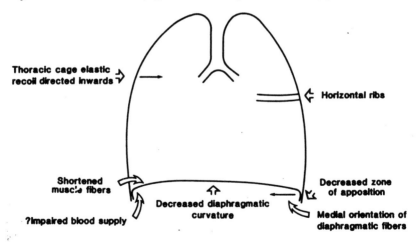

Figure 3: *The various detrimental effects of hyperinflation on respiratory muscle function. (From Tobin MJ. Respiratory muscles in disease. Clin Chest Med 1988; 9:263-286, with permission.)*

shortening of the diaphragm muscle fibers, thereby causing them to operate at a disadvantageous position on the length-tension curve. Hyperinflation also decreases diaphragmatic curvature and increases thoracic cage elastic recoil.[16] These, plus other factors, may collectively impair inspiratory muscle strength and/or endurance.

Although hyperinflation affects inspiratory muscle pressure (PI_{max}), some COPD patients also exhibit a decrease in expiratory muscle pressure (PE_{max}). Rochester and Braun[17] suggested that these patients have global respiratory muscle weakness possibly due to hypoxemia, hypercapnia, malnutrition, right heart failure with decreased blood supply to the respiratory muscles, corticosteroid-induced myopathy, or abnormalities in serum electrolytes. Accessory muscles of respiration may be recruited in an effort to assist respiratory function.

c. **Cystic fibrosis** Cough rather than dyspnea is the most prominent and constant symptom in patients with cystic fibrosis.[18] With progression of disease, dyspnea with daily activities frequently develops. Excessive airway secretions and airway reactivity lead to airflow obstruction and presumably contribute to breathlessness.

d. **Upper airway obstruction** The upper airway extends from the nasopharynx to the main carina and can be divided into extrathoracic (above the sternal notch) and intrathoracic (below the sternal notch) components. Dyspnea, wheezing, and/or stridor are the major symptoms of upper airway obstruction (UAO) and depend on the size and location of the obstruction in addition to the phase of respiration.[19] Generally, dyspnea and/or stridor will develop with exertion if the lesion reduces the diameter of the upper airway to about 8 mm.[20] An airway diameter of 5 mm or less at the site of obstruction will frequently produce inspiratory stridor and breathlessness at rest.[21] Typically, the patient prefers an upright posture because slight compression of the trachea may occur in the supine position due to the weight of mediastinal structures. Various conditions, or diseases, causing chronic dyspnea due to upper airway obstruction are listed in Table 3.

Enlarged adenoids and tonsils may be a problem for adolescents and young adults; dyspnea generally develops with physical exercise due to the added resistive load to breathing. Affected individuals may also experience obstructive sleep apnea and associated symptoms of

Table 3. Chronic Dyspnea Due to Major Causes of Upper Airway Obstruction

1. Enlarged adenoids and tonsils
2. Goiter
3. Parkinson's disease
4. Tracheal malignancy
5. Tracheal stenosis due to previous endotracheal intubation or tracheostomy
6. Vocal cord dysfunction (mimicking asthma)
7. Vocal cord paralysis (unilateral or bilateral)

snoring, poor sleep at night, and daytime hypersomnolence. Examination of the pharynx should identify enlarged lymphoid tissue.

Patients with a goiter can experience progressive dyspnea on exertion and wheezing that may be misdiagnosed as asthma.[22] Additional signs and symptoms of hyperthyroidism or hypothyroidism should be considered. An enlarged thyroid gland may be evident in the neck. Generally, there is a low-pitched stridor heard over the trachea and upper anterior chest, whereas the lung fields are clear. Non-surgical therapy can usually reduce the size of the goiter and improve respiratory symptoms.

Dyspnea can also be a symptom in Parkinson's disease.[23] In his original description of the disease that bears his name, Parkinson[24] noted that some patients "fetched their breath rather hard." Vincken et al.[25] reported that patients with Parkinson's disease can have UAO accompanied by changes in the voice and "running out of breath" when talking for long periods. The marked fluctuations in severity in the extrapyramidal manifestations can also be observed in respiratory function.[26] The UAO and associated dyspnea are reversible with levodopa therapy.[27]

Malignancies, both benign and malignant, can obstruct the trachea and lead to dyspnea.

The incidence of serious tracheal stenosis prior to the use of low-pressure endotracheal tube cuffs has been reported to be 3% to 20%.[28] In two prospective studies evaluating the low-pressure cuff, Stauffer et al.[29] and Colice et al.[30] showed that functionally significant tracheal stenosis was relatively uncommon with either endotracheal intubation or tracheostomy. If a stricture develops at the cuff site or stoma, dyspnea is the usual presenting symptom. A stenosis generally causes a fixed UAO,[31] although a variable, extrathoracic type has also been reported.[32]

Vocal cord dysfunction can mimic asthma attacks with associated symptoms of dyspnea and wheezing.[33] The majority of patients have been women between the ages of 20 and 40 years. The medical history often includes episodes of acute UAO leading to emergency hospitalization and even intubation. When asked to identify the site of airflow limitation, the patient typically points to the area of the vocal cords in front of the neck.[33] Laryngoscopy has demonstrated adduction of the anterior two-thirds of the vocal cords during an "attack," leaving only a small diamond-shaped opening at the back of the throat for passage of air. Psychological studies have suggested that vocal cord dysfunction presenting as asthma is a type of unconscious conversion disorder.[33] Speech therapy is indicated to reduce tension in the laryngeal musculature, whereas psychotherapy and supportive counseling are helpful in dealing with any underlying psychiatric disorder.

Unilateral or bilateral vocal cord paralysis may cause breathlessness, especially with exertion.[34,35] Generally, these lesions cause a variable, extrathoracic UAO as flow is diminished predominantly during inspiration. Diagnosis depends on laryngoscopy to directly examine vocal cord movement.

2. Parenchymal Lung Disease

Dyspnea is a major complaint among patients with interstitial lung disease (ILD), lung cancer, and pneumonia. Turner-Warwick et al.[36] reported 92% of patients with cryptogenic fibrosing alveolitis (also termed idiopathic pulmonary fibrosis in North America) present with dyspnea. Breathlessness is the initial complaint in 10% to 15% of patients with lung cancer, and occurs in up to 65% of patients at some point during the illness.[37] Also, dyspnea may occur in previously healthy individuals who develop pneumonia.

The breathing pattern in ILD is characterized by decreased tidal volume and increased frequency of respiration at rest and during exercise in response to the increased elastance.[38,39] It has been suggested previously that juxtacapillary (J) receptors are stimulated with interstitial inflammation and/or fibrosis and thereby contribute to the sense of breathlessness.[40] DiMarco et al.[38] speculated that vagal mechanisms and mechanoreceptors in the chest wall contribute to the altered breathing pattern in ILD patients. Burdon and colleagues[39] reported that the pattern of breathing adopted by patients with ILD during exercise (decreased peak inspiratory force and shorter duration of force development) actually may reduce the sensation of breathlessness. Mahler et al.[41] demonstrated that single-breath diffusing capacity ($D_L CO$) and exercise gas exchange are significantly related to clinical ratings of dyspnea in patients with diverse etiologies of ILD.

3. Pulmonary Vascular Disease

Dyspnea is the most common initial symptom in primary pulmonary hypertension, occurring in 60% of all patients.[42] Generally, dyspnea and fatigue are present for more than two years before the diagnosis is made. However, 98% of 187 patients with primary pulmonary hypertension experienced breathlessness at the time they were enrolled in the National Heart, Lung, and Blood Institute patient registry.[42] Patients with chronic pulmonary thromboemboli can experience similar complaints and, therefore, may be difficult to distinguish from other causes of pulmonary hypertension. Appropriate diagnosis is important because surgical therapy may produce remarkable improvement in patients with central thromboemboli causing vascular obstruction.[43]

Pulmonary function is variable in patients with pulmonary hypertension. Although most patients have normal lung volumes and flow rates, some exhibit a mild restrictive defect.[42] Diffusing capacity is usually reduced, and hypoxemia with chronic respiratory alkalosis often is present.[42] With even mild exertion, there is an excessive ventilatory response[44,45] (Figure 4). Possible receptor sites that mediate the sensation of dyspnea in pulmonary vascular disease include the pulmonary artery, right atrium, and right ventricle.[46-48]

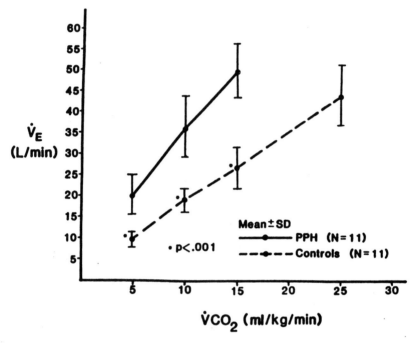

Figure 4: *Excessive ventilatory response to exercise ($\dot{V}_E$) in patients with primary pulmonary hypertension (PPH) compared to normal response in control subjects. (From D'Alonzo GE, Gianotti LA, Pohil RL, et al. Comparison of progressive exercise performance of normal subjects and patients with primary pulmonary hypertension. Chest 1987; 92:57-62, with permission.)*

4. Pleural Disease

The mechanism whereby fluid in the pleural space causes dyspnea is unclear. Pleural effusions act as space-occupying lesions and may compress the underlying lung and shift the heart and mediastinal structures to the contralateral side. Anthonisen and Martin[49] measured regional wash-out half-times during dynamic breathing in six patients with unilateral pleural effusions and found that dynamic ventilation was reduced in the lung regions underlying the effusion.

Removal of 1,000 to 1,500 mL of pleural fluid at a single thoracentesis generally provides improvement in breathlessness. However, the immediate change in lung function is modest. In nine patients who had 1,100 mL of fluid removed, the vital capacity increased by only 120 mL.[50] Light et al.[51] removed an average of 1,725 mL of pleural fluid from 14 patients and found that vital capacity improved only 480 mL at 24 hours after thoracentesis. Maximal improvement occurred several days later in some patients.[51] In addition, pulmonary gas exchange may actually worsen following thoracentesis. Brandstetter and Cohen[52] obtained arterial blood gases before and 20 minutes, 2 hours, and 24 hours after therapeutic thoracentesis in 16 patients. The mean arterial oxygen pressure (PaO_2) fell from 70 mmHg before the procedure to 61 mmHg and 64 mmHg at 20 minutes and 2 hours after thoracentesis, respectively. The physiological effects of the lateral decubitus position in unilateral pleural effusions are discussed in Chapter 5.

Thus, the symptom of dyspnea due to a pleural effusion does not appear to relate to usual parameters of lung function and/or gas exchange. It is possible that fluid in the pleural space may stimulate receptors in the chest wall and/or the airways in the underlying compressed lung to produce breathlessness. Removal of fluid may then reduce stimulation despite the minimal improvement in lung mechanics and possible decline in oxygenation.

5. Chest Wall Disease

The dominant feature of thoracic deformities and conditions which "load" the abdomen, e.g., obesity and pregnancy, is dyspnea on exertion without other respiratory symptoms such as cough and sputum production. All of the skeletal deformities of the thorax affect movement of the rib cage, while only a few appear to involve the diaphragm.[53] The major pathophysiological processes of thoracic deformities include the following: increased chest wall elastance; alveolar hypoventilation; and compression of lung leading to ventilation-perfusion ($\dot{V}/\dot{Q}$) mismatching and pulmonary hypertension.

In obesity, chest wall compliance is decreased due to accummulation of fat in and around the ribs, diaphragm, and abdomen. This requires increased respiratory work by the inspiratory muscles in order to expand and ventilate the lungs.[54] Naimark and Cherniack[55] demonstrated that total respiratory compliance in obese subjects fell substantially when they assumed the recumbent position, but this does not occur in normal, healthy individuals. Abdominal (gastric) pressure is increased with obesity and appears to be a linear function of body weight.[56] This increase serves to "load" the diaphragm by stretching its muscle fibers. Although an increase in length usually favors enhanced diaphragm function, pressure generation would be adversely affected by obesity if the preloaded diaphragm muscle fibers are stretched above optimal length.[54] Sampson and Grassino[57] described the development of respiratory muscle fatigue in massively obese subjects during CO_2 rebreathing. In addition, tidal breathing to upper lung zones in combination with perfusion to the bases can lead to $\dot{V}/\dot{Q}$ abnormalities in obesity.[58] These findings presumably account for hypoxemia, which is common in obese individuals.

In thoracic deformities and obesity, receptors in the chest wall, respiratory muscles, and/or joints of the thoracic cage may play a role in the genesis of dyspnea.

Dyspnea is a common complaint at some time during gestation and occurs in 60% to 70% of pregnant women.[59] It frequently begins in the first or second trimester of pregnancy prior to any increase in abdominal girth.[60-62] This observation suggests that mechanical factors are not a major cause for breathlessness. Cugell et al.[60] suggested that the increased drive to breathe induced by progesterone may explain the frequency of the symptom. Gilbert et al.[61,62] reported that the presence of dyspnea was correlated with low levels of arterial carbon dioxide pressure ($PaCO_2$) and that there was an enhanced ventilatory response to inhaled CO_2 in pregnant individuals who experience dyspnea. Although the exact mechanism of dyspnea in pregnancy is unclear, the sensation of breathlessness may be due to an increased ventilatory response that is inappropriate for the demand.

6. Respiratory Muscle Disease and/or Dysfunction

Respiratory muscle function can be affected by neuromuscular diseases (muscular dystrophy, amyotrophic lateral sclerosis, myasthenia gravis, and poliomyelitis), malnutrition, COPD, thyroid disease, and chronic primary fibromyalgia.[16,17,63-69] In some instances, diaphragm weakness may exist as an isolated finding without any detectable evidence outside of the respiratory system.[65] Also, global respiratory muscle weakness may develop naturally in healthy individuals who experience an upper respiratory tract infection.[66] Depending on the severity of weakness, dyspnea may be present at rest, particularly when supine, or only with certain physical activities.

Early in disease, PI_{max} and PE_{max} can be reduced even though FVC and FEV_1 are normal.[63] Weakness usually affects both inspiratory and expiratory muscles, although not always equally.[70] Gas exchange usually is well maintained in neuromuscular disease, although hypercapnia is likely when respiratory muscle strength falls to 30% of the predicted normal value.[71] Although the decrease in PI_{max} is caused in part by the loss of force generation by the muscles, instability of the chest wall muscles and rib cage-abdominal paradox may also contribute to weakness. In some patients, respiratory muscle weakness due to neuromuscular disease may go undetected until ventilatory failure and/or right heart failure are evident.

B. Cardiovascular

The precise stimulus for breathlessness in cardiovascular disease remains to be elucidated. The majority of cardiac conditions that contribute to dyspnea involve the left side of the heart and include ischemia, valvular disease, and myocardial dysfunction. Several factors may contribute to "cardiac dyspnea." The most widely stated explanation is an increase in left atrial, pulmonary venous, and pulmonary capillary pressures leading to transudation of fluid into the interstitium and ultimately into the alveolar spaces. The "congested" lungs exhibit a reduced compliance which adds to the work of breathing.[72] Presumably, J receptors are stimulated as fluid accumulates initially in the interstitium and triggers afferent impulses via the vagal nerve.[40] In addition, airway obstruction can develop in left ventricular failure due to congestion of bronchial vessels, peribronchial edema, reflex bronchoconstriction, and bronchial hyperresponsiveness.[73] These pathophysiological processes can obstruct airways and lead to "cardiac asthma."

However, not all patients with severe cardiac failure necessarily stop exercise due to breathlessness. Weber and Janicki[74] have observed that patients with chronic cardiac failure can walk 20 minutes without experiencing breathlessness despite having pulmonary occlusive wedge pressures of 30 mmHg or higher. These investigators suggested that dyspnea developed with anaerobic exercise and was related to the disproportionate increase in ventilation rather than elevated pulmonary venous pressure.[74]

Another possibility is that a reduced cardiac output response to exercise in patients with cardiovascular disease may contribute to dyspnea as a result of decreased oxygen delivery to respiratory muscles.[75] Additionally, but less frequently, causes of "cardiac dyspnea" include pericardial disease, left atrial myxoma, and intracardiac shunt.

C. Anemia

Anemia may contribute to breathlessness and general fatigue with activity. A low hemoglobin level leads to diminished oxygen-carrying capacity in the blood and places an added burden on the cardiovascular system to maintain adequate oxygen transport. Iron deficiency is probably the most common cause of anemia, especially in menstruating women.

D. Deconditioning

Dyspnea can occur in otherwise normal, healthy individuals as a result of exercise or other physical activities. High altitude or other environmental factors may contribute to this symptom. Such patients who seek medical evaluation for breathlessness may have normal cardiorespiratory function both at rest and with exertion. Apparently, the level of exercise ventilation, respiratory muscle output, and/or other physiological responses may be perceived by the individual as being excessive or inappropriate. In the deconditioned state, both cardiac and respiratory responses to submaximal exercise are higher than observed in those whose level of fitness is normal for their age.

E. Psychological Factors

Anxiety, depression, and other psychological factors may influence and/or magnify the sensation of dyspnea both at rest and with exertion. Some individuals with no evidence of organic disease may develop extreme anxiety when required to coordinate their breathing with the mechanics of a particular activity. These individuals may breathe normally at rest, but may breath-hold, hypoventilate, and/or hyperventilate with exercise, which subsequently leads to the experience of breathlessness.

III. Diagnosis

The basic principle of evaluating the patient with chronic dyspnea should be to begin with simple, non-invasive tests and then proceed to more complicated or invasive tests based on clues in the initial evaluation.[76]

A. History and Physical Examination

A careful history and physical examination are the key first steps in evaluating a patient who has chronic dyspnea. Since breathlessness is a subjective symptom experienced by almost everyone at some level of exertion, the critical first decision is whether the symptom is "normal" or represents disease. This decision should take into account the patient's age, general state of physical fitness and activity, change over time, comparison with appropriate peers, and other signs and symptoms of accompanying disease.

The patient's complaint of dyspnea should be related to a specific level of physical exertion since a patient who reduces his/her physical activity to avoid shortness of breath may stop reporting breathlessness. The physician or health-care provider should carefully question the patient about types of activities that provoke dyspnea, e.g., walking, climbing stairs, taking a shower, or carrying packages. Careful attention should be given to changes over months/years since chronic dyspnea frequently develops so gradually that the patient may not be aware of the onset of the disease in early stages. The spouse, other family members, or friends may be more aware of the change than the patient. The appropriate peer group for each patient should be used for comparison. Dyspnea in the young long-distance runner whose athletic performance decreases due to breathlessness may be just as important as in the older patient with emphysema who notes increasing difficulty playing golf. Change in dyspnea with body position may provide important clues (see Chapter 5). Attention also should be directed to other symptoms of disease in the systems commonly associated with dyspnea, e.g., angina due to coronary artery disease.

A careful physical examination can provide important clues to the origin of dyspnea and direct subsequent evaluation. Specific attention should focus on the examination of the heart and lungs, the two major organ systems associated with dyspnea. A heart murmur, gallop, increased heart size, peripheral edema, or distended jugular veins may indicate cardiac dysfunction. Left heart failure with pulmonary congestion may be manifest by signs of restrictive (interstitial/alveolar edema) and/or obstructive ("cardiac asthma") lung dysfunction. Obstructive airway disease may be indicated by diminished intensity of breath sounds, prolonged expiration or forced expiratory time, wheezing, and/or low diaphragmatic position with reduced excursion. Restrictive diseases may be suggested by tachypnea, an elevated diaphragm with normal respiratory excursion, end-inspiratory crackles, and/or signs of localized consolidation or effusion, e.g., dullness to percussion or changes in intensity of breath sounds. A loud pulmonary component of the second heart sound (P2), right ventricular heave, peripheral edema, and/or hepatojugular reflux may indicate right heart failure due to primary or secondary pulmonary hypertension. However, these changes are frequently subtle unless the disease is advanced.

In addition, clues to less common causes of dyspnea involving other organ systems may be manifest by the history and physical examination. A careful neurological examination may uncover evidence of muscle weakness or denervation which points to disease of the respiratory muscles as a possible cause of dyspnea.[77] Pallor or cyanosis may provide clues to anemia or hypoxemia, respectively, which may contribute to the patient's symptoms.

B. Basic Laboratory Tests

Laboratory evaluation of the dyspneic patient follows information derived from a careful history and physical examination. The following non-invasive "screening" tests are almost always indicated: chest radiograph; electrocardiogram; and a complete blood count. In addition, spirometry and a resting arterial blood gas measurement are essential first steps in the evaluation of suspected pulmonary dysfunction or disease.

Posterior-anterior and lateral chest radiographs are important in the evaluation of the patient with chronic dyspnea. These provide important information about both cardiac and respiratory diseases. Heart size, chamber enlargement, or signs of pulmonary congestion, e.g., cephalization of blood flow, perihilar haze, or interstitial or alveolar edema, may point to cardiac disease with concomitant left heart failure. Signs of restrictive lung diseases are commonly noted on chest radiographs, including parenchymal infiltrates (interstitial or alveolar) or pleural effusions. Abnormalities of the thoracic cage may be noted. Hyperinflated lung fields or bullous changes may indicate obstructive airway disease. Unilateral or bilateral diaphragmatic elevation may indicate involvement of the diaphragm from a neuromuscular process. Changes associated with pulmonary vascular disease often are absent or subtle, but may include hypovascular lung zones due to thromboembolic disease as well as pulmonary artery and/or right heart enlargement due to pulmonary hypertension. It should be emphasized, however, that a normal chest radiograph does not exclude disease processes associated with significant dyspnea. Diseases such as interstitial lung disease, pulmonary embolism, early left heart failure, or respiratory muscle disease may not produce significant or obvious radiographic abnormalities.

An electrocardiogram should be obtained and compared to previous records. This may provide important clues to disease of either the left or right heart, such as ischemia, arrhythmias, left or right atrial enlargement, right axis deviation, and right or left ventricular hypertrophy.

Routine blood tests should include a complete blood count to screen for anemia, which reduces the oxygen carrying capacity of the blood and provides a physiological stress which may contribute to dyspnea.

Subsequent testing depends on the collective results from a careful history and physical examination along with basic laboratory tests. In many cases, the cause of dyspnea will be apparent and a diagnosis can be made. In these cases, additional tests may be useful in confirming the diagnosis, staging the severity of a disease process, ruling out other concomitant diseases, or making decisions regarding therapy. In other circumstances, suspicion of certain diseases will narrow the range of diagnostic possibilities and allow additional tests to be selected to confirm specific etiologies. For example, signs and symptoms of thyrotoxicosis would lead to specific thyroid function tests.

In some cases, however, there may be few, if any, clues to diagnosis and the decision regarding subsequent testing is more difficult. Accordingly, if the physician believes that the patient's dyspnea has an organic basis, further evaluation should be directed primarily toward cardiopulmonary disorders.

C. Evaluation of Possible Pulmonary Causes

Lung diseases commonly produce breathlessness (Table 1) and should be considered in any patient with chronic dyspnea not obviously explained by another disease process. Lung diseases can be divided pathophysiologically into three categories: obstructive; restrictive; and vascular.

The initial and least invasive tests in evaluating a patient for pulmonary causes of dyspnea are pulmonary function studies, including spirometry, the flow-volume loop, and lung volume measurements.[78,79] These tests will be most useful in detecting and staging severity of obstructive, including upper airway, and restrictive lung diseases. These studies usually are normal in patients with pulmonary vascular disease, although some patients with pulmonary hypertension demonstrate a restrictive pattern on measurement of lung volumes.[80]

Spirometry provides important clues for the diagnosis of obstructive (reduced expiratory flow rates) and restrictive (reduced FVC with normal flow rates) lung diseases. Obstructive airway disease can be diagnosed by a decreased FEV_1/FVC ratio (typically, $< 70\%$) and/or a decreased FEF_{25-75}.[81,82] When asthma, or reactive airway disease, is suspected as the cause of dyspnea (or cough) and spirometric values are normal, testing for bronchodilator response may help to establish the diagnosis. An increase of $\geq 15\%$ in FEV_1 after an inhaled bronchodilator is the most widely used criterion to determine airway "reversibility."[83,84] Alternatively, bronchoprovocation testing with either methacholine or histamine can be used to diagnose airway "reactivity." A decrease of $\geq 20\%$ in FEV_1 after an inhaled bronchoconstrictor (methacholine or histamine) represents a "positive" test.[85]

The flow-volume loop is the best test to evaluate for UAO. In patients with obstructive sleep apnea, the flow-volume loop may reflect pharyngeal airway abnormalities characterized by "fluttering" or "sawtooth" configurations (Figure 5).[86,87] In patients with a goiter,

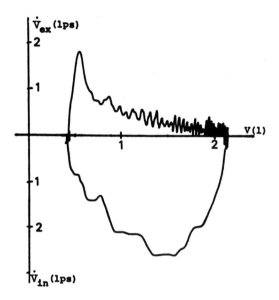

Figure 5: *Maximal flow-volume loop demonstrates "saw tooth" pattern particularly during expiration (upper portion of loop) in a patient with obstructive sleep apnea. This finding correlates with pharyngeal "fluttering" as observed during fiberoptic nasopharyngoscopy. (From Tammelin BR, Wilson AF, de Berry Borowiecki B, et al. Flow-volume curves reflect pharyngeal airway abnormalities in sleep apnea syndrome. Am Rev Respir Dis 1983; 128:712-715, with permission.)*

there is typically a fixed obstruction with a plateau on both inspiration and expiration; the airway diameter at the site of the obstruction does not change with the phase of respiration. In 24 of 27 patients (89%) with an extra-pyramidal disorder (essential action tremor or idiopathic Parkinson's disease), the flow-volume loop can show two abnormal patterns.[20] With "respiratory flutter," regular consecutive flow decelerations and accelerations were superimposed on the flow-volume loop (Figure 6). The second pattern consisted of irregular, abrupt changes in flow that dropped to zero, indicating intermittent airway closure (Figure 7). Patients with Parkinson's disease and UAO usually have decreased FEV_1 and FVC along with being more disabled than those without UAO.[20] Tumors in the proximal tracheobronchial tree can cause a fixed (Figure 8) or variable UAO. Although the characteristic finding in vocal cord dysfunction is abnormal inspiratory flow (Figure 9), both inspiratory and expiratory flow can be affected.

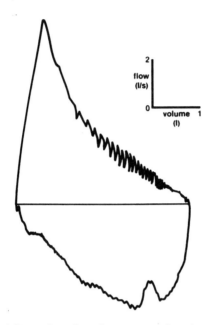

Figure 6: *Maximal flow-volume loop demonstrates "respiratory flutter" in a patient with Parkinson's disease. Regular and consecutive flow decelerations and accelerations were observed during expiration; endoscopy showed rhythmic changes in the glottic area due to alternating abduction and adduction of the vocal cords and supraglottic structures. (From Vincken WG, Gauthier SG, Dollfuss RE, et al. Involvement of upper-airway muscles in extrapyramidal disorders: a cause of airflow limitation. N Engl J Med 1984; 311:438-442, with permission.)*

Restrictive lung disease is defined by reduction in lung volumes (especially FVC and TLC). Expiratory flow rates may be variably affected. The pattern of lung volume change sometimes can be used to help distinguish the following various types of restrictive lung diseases: pleural, alveolar filling, interstitial, neuromuscular, and thoracic cage.[88,89] Obstructive airway diseases, such as asthma and COPD, typically produce an increase of certain lung volumes (particularly RV, FRC, and the RV/TLC ratio) in addition to the reduction in expiratory flow rates.

Measurement of the diffusing capacity for carbon monoxide can also provide useful information.[90] Reduction in the D_LCO may be a sensitive indicator of problems in pulmonary gas transfer, but is nonspecific since it may be decreased in emphysema, interstitial lung

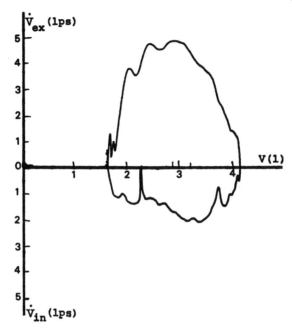

Figure 7: *Maximal flow-volume loop demonstrates irregular, abrupt changes in flow which often approaches zero (during inspiration) in a patient with Parkinson's disease. This finding represents intermittent airway closure. Endoscopy revealed irregular, jerky movements of the glottic and supraglottic structures. (From Vincken WG, Gauthier SG, Dollfuss RE, et al. Involvement of upper-airway muscles in extrapyramidal disorders: a cause of airflow limitation. N Engl J Med 1984; 311:438-442, with permission.)*

diseases, or pulmonary vascular diseases. In addition, the $D_L CO$ may be reduced in left heart failure with pulmonary congestion and anemia.

Measurement of arterial blood gases at rest is important to evaluate lung disease or acid-base abnormalities. The presence of hypoxemia and/or hypercapnia suggests problems with gas exchange or hypoventilation. Arterial pH and $PaCO_2$ values are useful to assess any acid-base disturbance.

Maximal inspiratory and expiratory mouth pressures are simple, non-invasive measurements that evaluate respiratory muscle strength and typically are reduced in the presence of respiratory muscle weakness.[63,91,92]

For the diagnosis of pulmonary vascular disease (pulmonary em-

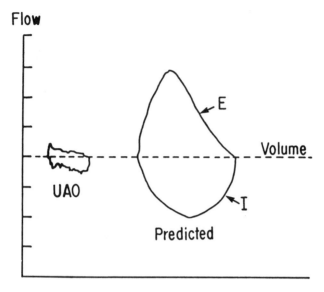

Figure 8: *Maximal flow-volume loop in a 61-year-old female with a squamous cell carcinoma obstructing the distal trachea and causing a fixed UAO. There is a plateau in flow during both expiration (E) and inspiration (I). The predicted normal flow-volume loop for this patient is shown on the right.*

boli, plexogenic pulmonary hypertension, or pulmonary veno-occlusive disease), one needs a high index of suspicion.[93] These diagnoses should be considered in any dyspneic patient whose symptoms are "unexplained" after the initial evaluation and testing. Ventilation-perfusion lung scanning is the usual first test to evaluate patients with suspected pulmonary vascular disease.[94] A normal $\dot{V}/\dot{Q}$ scan essentially excludes significant pulmonary vascular obstruction. Abnormalities in perfusion unmatched by ventilation suggest acute or chronic pulmonary embolic disease. Diffuse mottling or irregularity in perfusion may be seen in primary pulmonary hypertension. Ultimately, pulmonary angiography (and possibly right heart catheterization) may be necessary in evaluating the patient with suspected or known pulmonary vascular disease.

Pratter and coworkers[79] evaluated 85 consecutive patients who presented to a pulmonary specialty clinic with a primary complaint of dyspnea. Following the clinical impression obtained from history, physical examination, and chest roentgenogram, patients were subjected to additional diagnostic tests as necessary to establish what the

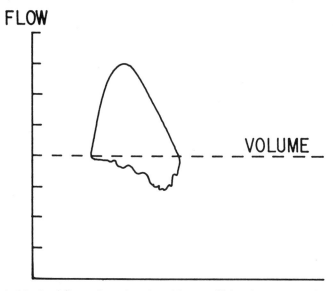

Figure 9: *Maximal flow-volume loop in a 22-year-old female patient with vocal cord dysfunction mimicking asthma. Typically, there is diminished inspiratory flow due to adduction of the anterior two-thirds of the vocal cords. This leaves only a small diamond-shaped opening at the back of the larynx for passage of air.*

authors considered a definitive diagnosis in each patient. The most common diagnoses were asthma (29%), COPD (14%), interstitial lung disease (14%), cardiomyopathy (11%), and upper airway disorders (8%) including postnasal drip and tracheal stenosis. The most frequently performed tests were spirometry, lung volumes, diffusing capacity, bronchodilator testing, and bronchoprovocation challenge testing in cases of suspected reactive airway disease. The clinical impression was found to be most accurate in diagnosing common disorders; less common diagnoses required additional diagnostic tests. Although the results of this study reflect both the referral pattern of patients to this subspecialty clinic and the diagnostic criteria set up by the authors, these results indicate that a diagnosis can be established in the majority of patients with an appropriate diagnostic approach.

D. Evaluation of Possible Cardiac Causes

In the patient with chronic dyspnea of possible cardiac origin, symptoms are likely due to left heart failure and concomitant pulmonary congestion. This may lead to either restrictive (interstitial and/or alveolar edema) or obstructive ("cardiac asthma") changes in lung function.[95] The initial evaluation of cardiac diseases as a cause for chronic dyspnea should focus on making a specific diagnosis, e.g., ischemia, valvular heart disease, or cardiomyopathy, and looking for evidence of pulmonary congestion, e.g., paroxysmal nocturnal dyspnea, orthopnea, or chest radiographic findings. When the diagnosis or the degree of cardiac involvement is uncertain, the physician or health-care provider should proceed with additional diagnostic tests in order of increasing complexity and level of invasiveness.

Echocardiography is very useful for evaluating chamber size, ventricular function, pericardial effusion, and valvular abnormalities. Radionuclide imaging techniques can also be helpful in this regard. Exercise stress testing may provide important information for diagnosing ischemic disease or arrhythmias during physical exertion. Ultimately, cardiac catheterization may be indicated to accurately diagnose and stage cardiac disease in selected patients.

E. Exercise Testing in Occult Causes of Chronic Dyspnea

Occasionally, patients are encountered with significant dyspnea but without evidence of sufficient pulmonary, cardiac, or other organ system disease on the initial evaluation to account for their symptom. The possibility of pulmonary vascular disease in this situation has been discussed already. Cardiopulmonary exercise testing may be extremely useful in distinguishing pulmonary, cardiac, or other causes of occult dyspnea and in assessing the degree to which the specific disease accounts for the patient's dyspnea.[96-99]

Exercise is a physiological stress on the oxygen transport system and requires integrated function of the lungs, pulmonary circulation, heart, systemic circulation, and skeletal muscles to provide sufficient energy needs to sustain physical activity. In general, the severity of dyspnea is related to the level of physical exertion for a given individual. Therefore, cardiopulmonary exercise testing in the laboratory is an ideal method for simulating the patient's symptom(s) and for evaluating specific physiological responses to increased work.

Cardiopulmonary exercise testing typically is performed on a cycle ergometer or treadmill in order to exercise large muscle groups to produce a high level of physiological stress. In the evaluation of chronic dyspnea, testing protocols typically employ incremental, progressive work loads to a symptom-limited maximum. An important part of testing is a careful evaluation and description of the signs and symptoms which develop during exercise and, ultimately, limit work performance. It is quite helpful to ask the patient at the end of the exercise test, "What limited you the most during exercise?" A complaint of chest pain, or angina, suggests the presence of ischemic heart disease. Intolerable dyspnea is most likely due to a respiratory disorder, although cardiovascular disease, deconditioning, anemia, and psychological conditions are other possibilities. The development of wheezing after exercise suggests exercise-induced bronchoconstriction. Ratings of perceived symptoms are very helpful in characterizing and quantifying different sensations, e.g., breathlessness and fatigue.[100,101]

Measurements obtained during cardiopulmonary exercise testing can range from simple to complex. The electrocardiogram can be used to measure heart rate and to evaluate for arrhythmias and ischemic changes. Minute ventilation ($\dot{V}_E$) can be measured to assess the ventilatory response to exercise. Monitoring expired gases for determination of $\dot{V}O_2$ and carbon dioxide elimination ($\dot{V}CO_2$) as well as other derived variables expands the diagnostic information. Measurement of arterial blood gases or oximetry during exercise reveals abnormalities in pulmonary gas exchange, such as exercise-induced hypoxemia and/or hypercapnia. In addition, combining arterial and expired gas measurements allows calculation of the alveolar-arterial oxygen difference and the dead space/tidal volume ratio.

Results of cardiopulmonary exercise testing provide important information about the organ system which limits exercise performance. Normal individuals have a substantial reserve in gas transport (O_2 and CO_2) capacity which allows for a large increase in physical work from resting levels. Since the heart and lungs are critical for oxygen transport, cardiopulmonary exercise testing is useful in detecting earlier stages of disease that reduce the maximal reserves in physiological function. The ventilatory reserve of the lungs can be assessed by comparing the peak exercise $\dot{V}_E$ to the measured (maximal voluntary ventilation, or MVV) or predicted ($FEV_1 \times 35-40$) maximal value for ventilation. Since the respiratory system generally does not limit exercise performance in normals, peak exercise $\dot{V}_E$ approximates 50%–80% of MVV in healthy individuals.[102] However, in patients with obstructive lung disease, "ventilatory limitation" may occur as reflected by the following: the level of $\dot{V}_E$ at a given work load exceeds the predicted range of values; and the peak exercise $\dot{V}_E$/MVV ratio is greater than 80% (Figure 10). In fact, in some

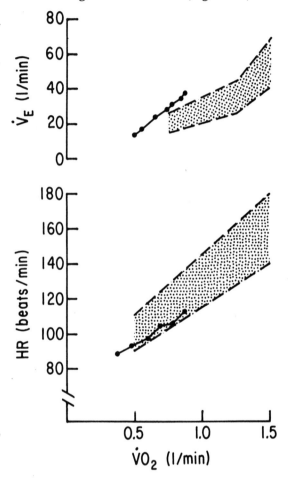

Figure 10: *Heart rate (HR) and minute ventilation ($\dot{V}_E$) responses to progressive, incremental exercise, as measured by oxygen consumption ($\dot{V}O_2$), in a 60-year-old male with severe obstructive airway disease. The HR response is at a low normal level (bottom panel), whereas $\dot{V}_E$ is above the normal range (upper panel). Peak HR was 114 beats/min, or 67% of the age-predicted maximal value (171 beats/min). Peak $\dot{V}_E$ was 37.7 l/min, or 90% of the maximal voluntary ventilation (42 l/min). These findings illustrate excessive ventilation and utilization of the ventilatory reserve and indicate "ventilatory limitation" to exercise.*

patients with severe COPD, the ratio may exceed 100%. In addition, pulmonary patients may demonstrate abnormalities in gas exchange during exercise, including hypoxemia and/or hypercapnia.

In contrast, cardiovascular performance potentially can limit maximal exercise performance in normal individuals. In healthy individuals, maximal cardiac output is approached at exhaustive exercise. Since stroke volume remains relatively constant above 40%–50% of peak $\dot{V}O_2$, normal individuals usually achieve 85% or more of the age-related, predicted maximal HR with exhaustive exercise.[96,97,102] In the patient with cardiac disease, "cardiovascular limitation" will be evident at low intensities of exercise. Thus, there will be a more rapid rise in HR at comparable levels of submaximal $\dot{V}O_2$, and maximal HR will be reached at a low level of $\dot{V}O_2$. Additional evidence of "cardiovascular limitation" to exercise is a low anaerobic threshold, i.e., lactic acidosis at a low work rate.

A more comprehensive discussion of exercise testing in the evaluation of pulmonary and cardiac diseases can be found in major textbooks.[96–99]

IV. Summary

Dyspnea is a common chronic complaint of patients with many different diseases. The evaluation of the patient with chronic dyspnea presents a number of diagnostic possibilities and pathways. Important clues can be found through a careful history and physical examination and the use of simple screening laboratory tests (chest radiograph, electrocardiogram, and complete blood count). From this information, the list of diagnostic possibilities usually can be narrowed considerably. In the patient without a readily apparent explanation for chronic dyspnea, attention should be directed toward the cardiac and pulmonary systems. A systematic approach starting with simple, non-invasive tests (pulmonary function and/or echocardiogram) and progressing to more technically complex and invasive ones, if needed, will frequently establish the diagnosis. Certain occult causes of chronic dyspnea (pulmonary embolism, pulmonary hypertension, respiratory muscle weakness, and deconditioning) should be considered when the diagnosis is not apparent. Cardiopulmonary exercise testing may be particularly helpful in evaluating the patient whose dyspnea is obscure after the initial evaluation and should be performed before attributing a patient's complaint of dyspnea to "non-organic" causes.

References

1. Marshall R, Stone RW, Christie RV. The relationship of dyspnoea to respiratory effort in normal subjects, mitral stenosis and emphysema. Clin Sci 1954; 13:625- 631.
2. Mahler DA, Weinberg DH, Wells CK, et al. The measurement of dyspnea: contents, interobserver agreement, and physiologic correlates of two new clinical indexes. Chest 1984; 85:751-758.
3. Killian KJ, Campbell EJM. Dyspnea. In: Roussos C, Macklem PT (eds). The Thorax: Part B. New York, Marcel Dekker, Inc., 1985; 787-828.
4. Smolensky MH, Barnes PJ, Reinberg A, et al. Chronobiology and asthma. I. Day-night differences in bronchial patency and dyspnea and circadian rhythm dependencies. J Asthma 1986; 23: 321-343.
5. Barnes P, FitzGerald G, Brown M, et al. Nocturnal asthma and changes in circulating epinephrine, histamine, and cortisol. N Engl J Med 1980; 303:263-267.
6. Dethlefsen U, Repges R. Ein neues therapieprinzys bei nachtlichem asthma. Med Klin 1985; 80:44-47.
7. Rubinfeld AR, Pain MCF. Perception of asthma. Lancet 1976; i:882-884.
8. Burdon JGW, Juniper EF, Killian KJ, et al. The perception of breathlessness in asthma. Am Rev Respir Dis 1982; 126:825-828.
9. Peiffer C, Marsac J, Lockhart A. Chronobiological study of the relationship between dyspnoea and airway obstruction in symptomatic subjects. Clin Sci 1989; 77:237-244.
10. Janson-Bjerklie S, Schnell S. Effect of peak flow information on patterns of self-care in adult asthma. Heart Lung 1988; 17:543-549.
11. Tangri S, Woolf CR. The breathing pattern in chronic obstructive lung disease during the performance of some common daily activities. Chest 1973; 63:126-127.
12. Celli BR, Rassulo J, Make BJ. Dyssynchronous breathing during arm but not leg exercise in patient with chronic airflow obstruction. N Engl J Med 1986; 314:1485-1490.
13. Cherniack RM. The oxygen consumption and efficiency of the respiratory muscles in health and emphysema. J Clin Invest 1959; 38:494-499.
14. Milic-Emili G, Peter JM. Mechanical efficiency of breathing. J Appl Physiol 1960; 15:359-362.
15. Rochester DF, Arora NS, Braun NMT, et al. The respiratory muscles in chronic obstructive pulmonary disease (COPD). Bull Eur Physiopathol Respir 1979; 15:951-975.
16. Tobin MJ. Respiratory muscles in disease. Clin Chest Med 1988; 9:263-286.
17. Rochester DF, Braun NMT. Determinants of maximal inspiratory pres-

sure in chronic obstructive pulmonary disease. Am Rev Respir Dis 1985; 132:42-47.

18. Wood RE, Boat TF, Doershuk CF. Cystic fibrosis. Am Rev Respir Dis 1976; 113:833-865.
19. Acres JC, Kryger MH. Upper airway obstruction. Chest 1981; 80:207-211.
20. Al-Bazzaz F, Grillo HC, Kazemi H. Responses to exercise in upper airway obstruction. Am Rev Respir Dis 1975; 111:631-640.
21. Geffin B, Grillo HC, Cooper JD, et al. Stenosis following tracheostomy for respiratory care. JAMA 1971; 216:1984-1988.
22. Karbowitz SR, Edelman LB, Nath S, et al. Spectrum of advanced upper airway obstruction due to goiters. Chest 1985; 87:18-20.
23. Nugent CA, Harris HW, Cohen J, et al. Dyspnea as a symptom in Parkinson's syndrome. Am Rev Tuberc 1958; 78:682-691.
24. Parkinson J. An Assay on the Shaking Palsy. London, Whittingham & Rowland, 1817.
25. Vincken WG, Gauthier SG, Dollfuss RE, et al. Involvement of upper-airway muscles in extrapyramidal disorders: a cause of airflow limitation. N Engl J Med 1984; 311:438-442.
26. Ilson J, Braun N, Fahn S. Respiratory fluctuations in Parkinson's disease (abstract). Neurology 1983; 33 (suppl 2):113.
27. Vincken WG, Darauay CM, Cosio MG. Reversibility of upper airway obstruction after levodopa therapy in Parkinson's disease. Chest 1989; 96:210-212.
28. Pearson FG, Goldberg M, DaSilva AJ. A prospective study of tracheal injury complicating tracheostomy with cuffed tube. Ann Otol Rhinol Laryngol 1968; 77:867-872.
29. Stauffer JL, Olson DE, Petty TL. Complications and consequences of endotracheal intubation and tracheostomy. Am J Med 1981; 20:65-76.
30. Colice GL, Stukel TA, Dain B. Laryngeal complications of prolonged intubation. Chest 1989; 96:877-884.
31. Kryger M, Bode F, Antic R, et al. Diagnosis of obstruction of the upper and central airways. Am J Med 1976; 61:85-93.
32. Calhoun WJ, Davis GS. Variable tracheal stenosis related to body position. Chest 1984; 86:87-89.
33. Christopher KL, Wood RP, Eckert RC, et al. Vocal cord dysfunction presenting as asthma. N Engl J Med 1983; 308:1566-1570.
34. Cormier Y, Kashima H, Summer W, et al. Upper airways obstruction with bilateral vocal cord paralysis. Chest 1979; 75:423-427.
35. Cormier Y, Kashima H, Summer W, et al. Airflow in unilateral vocal cord paralysis before and after Teflon injection. Thorax 1978; 33:57-61.
36. Turner-Warwick M, Burrows B, Johnson A. Crytogenic fibrosing alveolitis: clinical features and their influence on survival. Thorax 1980; 35: 171-180.
37. Reuben DB, Mor V. Dyspnea in terminally ill cancer patients. Chest 1986; 89:234-236.
38. DiMarco AF, Kelsen SG, Cherniack NS, et al. Occlusion pressure and

breathing pattern in patients with interstitial lung disease. Am Rev Respir Dis 1983; 127:425-430.

39. Burdon JGW, Killian KJ, Jones NL. Pattern of breathing during exercise in patients with interstitial lung disease. Thorax 1983; 38:778-784.

40. Rebuck AS, Slutsky AS. Control of breathing in diseases of the respiratory tract and lungs. In: Cherniack NS, Widdicombe JG (eds). Handbook of Physiology, Section 3: The Respiratory System. Bethesda, American Physiological Society, 1986; 771-791.

41. Mahler DA, Harver A, Rosiello RA, et al. Measurement of respiratory sensation in interstitial lung disease: evaluation of clinical dyspnea ratings and magnitude scaling. Chest 1989; 96:767-771.

42. Rich S, Dantzker DR, Ayres SM, et al. Primary pulmonary hypertension. Ann Intern Med 1987; 107: 216-223.

43. Moser KM, Daily PO, Peterson K, et al. Thromboendarterectomy for chronic, major-vessel thromboembolic pulmonary hypertension. Ann Intern Med 1987; 107:560-565.

44. Janicki JS, Weber KT, Likoff MJ, et al. Exercise testing to evaluate patients with pulmonary vascular disease. Am Rev Respir Dis 1984; 129(suppl):S93-S95.

45. D'Alonzo GE, Gianotti LA, Pohil RL, et al. Comparison of progressive exercise performance of normal subjects and patients with primary pulmonary hypertension. Chest 1987; 92:57-62.

46. Harrison TR, Harrison WG Jr, Calhoun JA, et al. Congestive heart failure. XVII. The mechanism of dyspnea on exertion. Arch Intern Med 1932; 50:690-720.

47. Uchida Y. Tachypnea after stimulation of afferent cardiac sympathetic nerve fibers. Am J Physiol 1976; 230:1003-1007.

48. Jones PW, Huszczuk A, Wasserman K. Cardiac output as a controller of ventilation through changes in right ventricular load. J Appl Physiol 1982; 53:218-224.

49. Anthonisen NR, Martin RR. Regional lung function in pleural effusion. Am Rev Respir Dis 1977; 116:201-207.

50. Brown NE, Zamel N, Aberman A. Changes in pulmonary mechanics and gas exchange following thoracentesis. Chest 1978; 74:540-542.

51. Light RW, Stansbury DW, Brown SE. The relationship of pleural pressures and changes in pulmonary function following therapeutic thoracentesis. Am Rev Respir Dis 1986; 133:658-661.

52. Brandstetter RD, Cohen RP. Hypoxemia after thoracentesis. A predictable and treatable condition. JAMA 1979; 242:1060-1061.

53. Bergofsky EH. Thoracic deformities. In: Roussos C, Macklem PT (eds). The Thorax, Part B. New York, Marcel Dekker, Inc., 1985; 941-978.

54. Sharp JT. The chest wall and respiratory muscles in obesity, pregnancy, and ascites. In: Roussos C, Macklem PT (eds). The Thorax, Part B. New York, Marcel Dekker, Inc., 1985; 999-1021.

55. Naimark A, Cherniack RM. Compliance of the respiratory system in health and obesity. J Appl Physiol 1960; 15:377-382.

56. Hackney JD, Crane MG, Collier CC, et al. Syndrome of extreme obesity

and hypoventilation: studies of etiology. Ann Intern Med 1959; 51:541-552.

57. Sampson MG, Grassino A. Diaphragmatic muscle fatigue in the massively obese. Am Rev Respir Dis 1981; 123 (suppl):183.

58. Holley HS, Milic-Emili J, Becklake MR, et al. Regional distribution of pulmonary ventilation and perfusion in obesity. J Clin Invest 1967; 46:475-481.

59. Prowse CM, Gaensler EA. Respiratory and acid-base changes during pregnancy. Anesthesiology 1965; 26:381-392.

60. Cugell DW, Frank NR, Gaensler EA, et al. Pulmonary function in pregnancy. I. Serial observations in normal women. Am Rev Tuberc 1953; 67:568-597.

61. Gilbert R, Epifano L, Auchincloss JH Jr. Dyspnea of pregnancy: a syndrome of altered respiratory control. JAMA 1962; 182:1073-1077.

62. Gilbert R, Auchincloss JH Jr. Dyspnea of pregnancy: clinical and physiological observations. Am J Med Sci 1966; 252:270-276.

63. Black LF, Hyatt RE. Maximal static respiratory pressures in generalized neuromuscular disease. Am Rev Respir Dis 1971; 103:641-650.

64. Mier A, Brophy C, Wass JAH, et al. Reversible respiratory muscle weakness in hyperthyroidism. Am Rev Respir Dis 1989; 139:529-533.

65. Mier-Jedrzejowicz A, Brophy C, Moxham J, et al. Assessment of diaphragm weakness. Am Rev Respir Dis 1988; 137:877-883.

66. Mier-Jedrzejowicz A, Brophy C, Green M. Respiratory muscle weakness during upper respiratory tract infections. Am Rev Respir Dis 1988; 138:5-7.

67. Smith PEM, Calverly MB, Edwards RHT, et al. Practical problems in the respiratory care of patients with muscular dystrophy. N Engl J Med 1987; 316:1197-1205.

68. Vicken W, Elleker MG, Cosio MG. Determinants of respiratory muscle weakness in stable chronic neuromuscular disorders. Am J Med 1987; 82:53-58.

69. Caidahl K, Lurie M, Blake B, et al. Dyspnoea in chronic primary fibromyalgia. J Intern Med 1989; 226:265-270.

70. Rochester DF. Tests of respiratory muscle function. Clin Chest Med 1988; 9:249-261.

71. Braun NMT, Arora NS, Rochester DF. Respiratory muscle and pulmonary function in polymyositis and other proximal myopathies. Thorax 1983; 38:616-623.

72. Flick MR. Pulmonary edema and acute lung injury. In: Murray JF, Nadel JA (eds). Textbook of Respiratory Medicine. Philadelphia, W.B. Saunders, 1988; 1359-1409.

73. Cabanes LR, Weber SN, Matran R, et al. Bronchial hyperresponsiveness to methacholine in patients with impaired left ventricular function. N Engl J Med 1989; 320:1317-1322.

74. Weber KT, Janicki JS. Lactate production during maximal and submaximal exercise in patients with chronic cardiac failure. J Am Coll Cardiol 1985; 6:717-724.

75. Macklem PT. Respiratory muscles: the vital pump. Chest 1980; 78:753-758.
76. Moser KM. Evaluation of patients with acute or chronic dyspnea. In: Moser KM, Spragg RG (eds). Respiratory Emergencies. C.V. Mosby Co. St. Louis, 1982; 214-230.
77. Weiner WJ. Respiratory Dysfunction in Neurologic Disease. Mt. Kisco, NY, Futura Publishing Co., 1980; 1-336.
78. Tisi GM. Pulmonary Physiology in Clinical Medicine, 2nd Edition. Baltimore, Williams & Wilkins, 1983; 1-287.
79. Pratter MR, Curley FJ, Dubois J, et al. Cause and evaluation of chronic dyspnea in a pulmonary disease clinic. Arch Intern Med 1989; 149:2277-2282.
80. Horn M, Ries A, Neveu C, et al. Restrictive ventilatory pattern in precapillary pulmonary hypertension. Am Rev Respir Dis 1983; 128:163-165.
81. Dosman J, Bode F, Urbanetti J, et al. The use of helium-oxygen mixture during maximum expiratory flow to demonstrate obstruction in small airways in smokers. J Clin Invest 1975; 55:1090-1099.
82. Gilbert R, Auchincloss H Jr. The interpretation of the spirogram. How accurate is it for 'obstruction'? Arch Intern Med 1985; 145:1635-1639.
83. Ries AL. Response to bronchodilators. In: Clausen JL, Zarins LP (eds). Pulmonary Function Testing Guidelines and Controversies: Equipment, Methods, and Normal Values. New York, Academic Press, 1982; 215-221.
84. Light RW, Conrad SA, George RB. The one best test for evaluating effects of bronchodilator therapy. Chest 1977; 72:512-516.
85. Braman SS, Corrao WM. Bronchoprovocation testing. Clin Chest Med 1989; 10:165-176.
86. Walsh RE, Michaelson ED, Harkleroad LE, et al. Upper airway obstruction in obese patients with sleep disturbance and somnolence. Ann Intern Med 1972; 76:185-192.
87. Tammelin BR, Wilson AF, de Berry Borowiecki B, et al. Flow-volume curves reflect pharyngeal airway abnormalities in sleep apnea syndrome. Am Rev Respir Dis 1983; 128:712-715.
88. Ries AL. Measurement of lung volumes. Clin Chest Med 1989; 10:177-186.
89. Ries AL, Clausen JL. Lung volumes. In: Wilson AF (ed). Pulmonary Function Testing Indications and Interpretations. Orlando, Grune & Stratton, 1985;69-85.
90. Ayers LN. Carbon monoxide diffusing capacity. In: Wilson AF (ed). Pulmonary Function Testing Indications and Interactions. Orlando, Grune & Stratton, 1985;137-151.
91. Black LF, Hyatt RE. Maximal respiratory pressures: normal values and relationship to age and sex. Am Rev Respir Dis 1969; 99:696-702.
92. Clausen JL. Maximal inspiratory and expiratory pressures. In: Clausen JL, Zarins LP (eds). Pulmonary Function Testing Guidelines and Controversies. New York, Academic Press, 1982;187-191.

93. Moser KM. Pulmonary embolism. Am Rev Respir Dis 1977; 115:829-852.
94. Alderson PO, Martin EC. Pulmonary embolism: diagnosis with multiple imaging modalities. Radiology 1987; 164:297-312.
95. Ries AL, Gregoratos G, Friedman PJ, et al. Pulmonary function tests in the detection of left heart failure: correlation with pulmonary wedge pressures. Respiration 1986; 49:241-250.
96. Wasserman K, Hansen JE, Sue DY. Principles of exercise testing and interpretation. Philadelphia, Lea & Febriger, 1987.
97. Jones NL. Clinical Exercise Testing, 3rd Edition. Philadelphia, W.B. Saunders Co., 1988.
98. Ries AL. The role of exercise testing in pulmonary diagnosis. Clin Chest Med 1987; 8:81-89.
99. Froelicher VF. Exercise and the Heart, 2nd Edition. Chicago, Year Book Medical Publishers, Inc., 1987.
100. Borg GAV. Psychophysical bases of perceived exertion. Med Sci Sports Exerc 1982; 14:377-381.
101. Mahler DA. Dyspnea: diagnosis and management. Clin Chest Med 1987; 8:215-230.
102. Hansen JE, Sue DY, Wasserman K. Predicted values for clinical exercise testing. Am Rev Respir Dis 1984; 129(suppl):S49-S55.

Chapter 7

Coping and Self-Care Strategies

Virginia Kohlman-Carrieri and Susan Janson-Bjerklie

From *Dyspnea*, edited by Donald A. Mahler, M.D., © 1990, Futura Publishing Company, Inc., Mount Kisco, NY.

I. Introduction

The symptom of dyspnea has an impact on the life of an individual that goes far beyond the understanding of most health-care providers. Dyspnea is a pervasive and disruptive symptom that causes loss of social interaction, self-esteem, occupational pursuits, mobility, creative endeavors, and recreational and social activities. A patient with dyspnea is required to make significant changes in his/her life-style and social/personal situation. Coping with this distressful symptom becomes the focus of existence and daily life for many patients. Improving a person's ability to cope with the illness should be a major treatment goal and is thought to be as important as treating the physical aspects of the disease.[1,2]

Health-care providers often have viewed dyspnea as just one more consequence of chronic pulmonary disease, not worthy of attention in its own right. Too often in the past, the focus has been on the correct diagnosis and treatment of the disease rather than the symptom. When the disease has received maximal medical and pharmacological treatment, patients often are told that "we have done all we can," and that they must endure and live with the symptoms accompanying the illness. This attitude can foster hopelessness and powerlessness when patients are led to believe that nothing more can be done and there is no hope for disease remission. However, the symptom of dyspnea is treatable (see Chapter 8). Patients can learn that there are strategies that can be used to decrease the distress of the symptom and the devastating effect of the illness on the psychological and social aspects of life.

The health-care provider and patient may not be able to decrease the intensity of the symptom, but together they can modulate the distress of the symptom. Symptom characteristics often are more important for the patient than the physiology of the disease itself.[3] The frequency, permanency, predictability, visibility, and social meaning of a symptom are just some of the characteristics that determine the amount of distress a person experiences and the impact that the symptom has on a patient's mood, activities of daily living, and quality of life. The temporal pattern of dyspnea is important since the frequency of episodes of severe dyspnea probably correlates with the degree of experienced distress and the disruption of life. Variability of symptom episodes produces erratic patterns of peaks and valleys of intensities. In patients with chronic dyspnea, a sudden or insidious rise in intensity due to a respiratory infection or physical exertion can produce severe dyspnea superimposed on the baseline severity. These episodic variations are distressing and require different coping strategies.

Another important symptom dimension is predictability. The unexpected or unanticipated episodes of acute dyspnea that sometimes occur in asthma produce uncertainty and panic. The meaning of dyspnea to the patient and the visibility of associated behaviors bring this symptom into a social and work context. Patients with chronic severe dyspnea experience loss of functional ability, social isolation, and marked changes in work capability that lead to loss of self-esteem. The experience of dyspnea by the patient or the meaning of the symptom to the person is related to the success in coping with dyspnea.

II. Theoretical Perspectives on Coping

A theoretical perspective for understanding coping responses of patients with dyspnea is provided by Lazarus and Folkman,[4] who hypothesize that individuals and their environments reciprocally affect each other. Coping is described as constantly changing cognitive and behavioral efforts used to manage external and internal demands that are appraised as exceeding the person's resources. Coping is goal-directed and elicited when the individual cognitively appraises an event as harmful, beneficial, threatening, or challenging. The appraisal is thought to generate emotions which influence the coping process. Coping is viewed not as a modifying variable, but as a mediator of emotional responses arising during an encounter and changing the original appraisal and associated emotion in some way.[5]

The process of coping includes primary appraisal, which is the assessment of a stressful situation as harmful or challenging, and secondary appraisal, the assessment of whether resources are available to meet the demands imposed by the stressful event. The stressful situation in chronic lung disease is the increase in dyspnea intensity and associated distress. The perception of the symptom and possible ways of decreasing it determine how patients will cope. For example, if past experience has led those with chronic lung disease to develop a repertoire of strategies that can be used to ameliorate the dyspnea, then they can cope successfully and theoretically experience less distress and anxiety.

Variables or factors that modify primary appraisal and symptom intensity include the following: patient characteristics, such as age, knowledge, and beliefs; regimen requirements; disease and symptom characteristics; available social support; and patient-practitioner relationships. The impact of these modifying factors affects the coping strategies and patterns that patients develop and use.[6] Using available literature, we have developed a model specifically for the symptom of dyspnea, outlining those variables or antecedents that may affect primary appraisal, self-care, and coping strategies, which in turn alter the experience of dyspnea.[7]. Antecedent variables are categorized into personal, illness, and situational dimensions (Table 1).

Table 1. Variables Related to Dyspnea

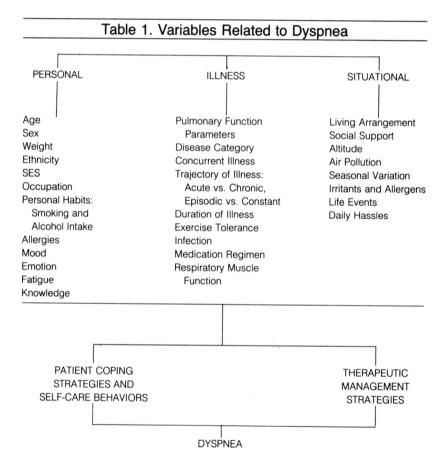

PERSONAL	ILLNESS	SITUATIONAL
Age	Pulmonary Function	Living Arrangement
Sex	Parameters	Social Support
Weight	Disease Category	Altitude
Ethnicity	Concurrent Illness	Air Pollution
SES	Trajectory of Illness:	Seasonal Variation
Occupation	Acute vs. Chronic,	Irritants and Allergens
Personal Habits:	Episodic vs. Constant	Life Events
Smoking and	Duration of Illness	Daily Hassles
Alcohol Intake	Exercise Tolerance	
Allergies	Infection	
Mood	Medication Regimen	
Emotion	Respiratory Muscle	
Fatigue	Function	
Knowledge		

PATIENT COPING
STRATEGIES AND
SELF-CARE BEHAVIORS

THERAPEUTIC
MANAGEMENT
STRATEGIES

DYSPNEA

This framework is only a beginning model. Additional critical variables related to the development and perception of dyspnea need to be identified and studied systematically.

Theorists differentiate between self-care and coping (see Table 2). Self-care is the repetitive use of strategies that have been proven effective in the past. Coping is a response to a new or different situation that requires modification of formerly effective strategies or the development of entirely new ones. Such a situation can occur in a patient with chronic lung disease when a sudden episode of dyspnea develops in a new environment or under conditions where resources (secondary appraisal) may not be available. The potential for harm (primary appraisal) appears great to the patient under such circumstances, especially when previously used strategies that were once effective no longer work. To cope, the patient must devise new strategies using new resources to get through the situation successfully. These episodes become pivotal experiences that shape future coping behavior for the patient.

III. Coping Strategies

Coping can be categorized into problem-focused, emotion-focused or mixed coping.[8] Problem-focused coping involves efforts that change the situation, e.g., making a plan of action and following

---

Table 2. Summary of Definitions of Coping

Self-Care: Repetitive use of strategies that have proven effective in the past.

Coping: Constantly changing cognitive and behavioral efforts used to manage external and internal demands that are appraised as exceeding the person's resources. Coping is a response to a new or different situation that requires modification of old strategies or development of new ones.

Primary Appraisal: The evaluation of the significance of the event as irrelevant, benign or stressful. If stressful, appraisal includes whether there is harm or loss, threat, or if it is a challenge.

Secondary Appraisal: The evaluation of what coping resources and options the individual has available.

Problem-Focused Coping: Efforts that change the situation.

Emotion-Focused Coping: Efforts to reduce psychological tension.

it, whereas emotion-focused coping involves efforts to reduce psychological tension, e.g., trying to look on the bright side of things or trying to relax. Coping has also been discussed as episodic, referring to strategies used in a particular situation, or adaptational, which are long-term changes in self-care. Self-care or coping strategies also can be categorized into cognitive and behavioral strategies. Cognitive strategies involve attempts to modify thought processes, thinking, and knowledge in order to attenuate a symptom. Behavioral strategies can be used to terminate a stressful event, make it less probable, make it less intense, or change the duration or timing of a stressor or symptom.[9]

Recent research indicates that patients use many types of coping strategies concurrently or use strategies that may have more than one coping function, depending on the psychological context in which it occurs. Seeking social support, for example, can serve both problem- and emotion-focused functions. Typical coping behaviors are categorized into such strategies as confrontive coping, distancing, self-control, seeking social support, problem-solving, and positive reappraisal; these factors represent the major scales in the Ways of Coping Questionnaire.[10] These strategies employed by a healthy population cannot be generalized to seriously ill people coping with a symptom such as dyspnea. However, it has been observed previously that such strategies like those listed above have been used by patients with various pulmonary diseases who experience dyspnea.[11]

Three general intervention strategies have been described recently that can be used to promote effective coping behavior and enhance the patient's quality of life.[12] The first strategy is to minimize the psychophysiological impact on the patient's lifestyle by teaching him/her breathing strategies and appropriate use of stress management and self-management skills. The second strategy is described as assessing and providing appropriate coping mechanisms and social support, including family assistance, counseling, and structured support groups. The third strategy involves increasing the patient's sense of hope, optimism, and self-esteem.

To help patients cope with chronic dyspnea that varies in intensity, the approach should be individualized to the patient's historical profile, episode characteristics, and personal responses. These strategies for coping can be targeted to specific kinds of episodes. For example, the patient with COPD who primarily experiences an acute increase in dyspnea with physical exertion can learn to anticipate the activity, use specific breathing techniques, and move slower. Another example is the patient who experiences anxiety or panic attacks either before or in association with dyspneic episodes. Those who believe their dyspnea is triggered by anxiety or panic may be helped by being taught to use a relaxation, panic-control strategy. Self-care or adaptational strategies that have been effective in the past for other patients can be discussed individually or in structured pulmonary rehabilitation programs.

IV. Effective Self-Care and Coping Strategies

A. Position

A change in body position during an acute attack of dyspnea may decrease dyspnea for some patients. During an acute episode of dyspnea, standing still, finding a "breathing station" to sit or lean on, or just being "motionless," "keeping still," or "staying quiet" are behaviors that patients have described. A relief position for patients is the leaning forward position, either standing or sitting. If a patient is standing, he/she can lean forward with his/her forearms on a chair or another tall object, with shoulders and arms relaxed. While seated, the patient can lean forward with his/her arms supported by a table, the arms of a chair, or his/her knees. The patient typically bends forward at the waist while bearing weight on his/her hands or elbows for support; the hands and shoulders are relaxed while the back is straight. Leaning forward on pillows placed on a desk or table also may be comfortable. The head-down position and the leaning forward position have been found to decrease dyspnea.[13] This postural relief is thought to be due to an increase in the mechanical advantage, or length-tension relationship, of the diaphragm. Abdominal contents can push up on the diaphragm and increase the resting length of the diaphragm, thereby improving its ability to generate force.[13]

Patients with chronic lung disease find the "best" position to reduce dyspnea on their own and should be encouraged to assume this position when dyspnea develops. It is important to recognize that patients usually assume the position that is most comfortable and provides the most physiological benefit.[14]

B. Pursed-Lips Breathing and Paced Breathing

Either during acute episodes or with constant chronic dyspnea, patients may experience less dyspnea with the use of pursed-lips breathing (PLB). In the past, exhalation through pursed lips was thought to modify dyspnea by raising the pressure in the airways, simulating positive end-expiratory pressure and providing internal stability to the airways to prevent early airway closure. More likely, the decrease in reported dyspnea is due to the associated decrease in respiratory rate and corresponding increase in tidal volume,[15,16] leading to an increase in oxygen saturation.[17] Patients often adopt this strategy spontaneously. If they are not using pursed-lips breathing already, patients should be instructed to inhale through the nose or mouth very slowly and deeply, purse their lips like they are going to whistle, and exhale slowly through pursed lips, taking twice as long to exhale as to inhale. Inhalation should occur during rest, with exhalation through pursed lips during actual exertion of a task. If the patient is unable to purse his/her lips, he/she can be instructed to breathe through a fist held up to the mouth. Even patients who previously have used pursed-lips breathing may not understand the rationale for the maneuver and need instruction in the correct technique. Repeated demonstration and practice to minimize hyperventilation and to increase the efficiency and timing of pursing the lips on exhalation and with the effort of a task is very important. Patients should be instructed not to hyperventilate by either breathing too deeply or exhaling too long or too hard.

Pursed-lips breathing should be combined with paced breathing, that is, resting with inspiration and exhaling with the activity such as walking, climbing the stairs, or bending to tie a shoe. Paced breathing means pacing the patient's work to his/her capacity and maintaining a controlled breathing pattern of exhalation when the effort or work is being done. Although the benefit of PLB for reducing breathlessness is not well documented in scientific studies, patients generally report less dyspnea and describe a feeling of control of their breathing. It must be emphasized that the patient needs extensive practice, demonstration, and repeated demonstration with all types of tasks including lifting, bending, walking, and stair climbing. Reinforcement of PLB should continue at patient visits with appropriate questions about when the patient is using PLB, the technique used, and whether the technique is helping to reduce dyspnea.

C. Diaphragmatic or Abdominal Breathing

Diaphragmatic or abdominal breathing means active use of the diaphragm rather than accessory muscles during inspiration. This technique is most helpful for patients who demonstrate at least minimal diaphragmatic excursion on physical examination. It is unlikely to be effective for the patient with a low, "fixed" diaphragm; however, some patients still find this type of breathing to be relaxing and calming. It also may be useful during routine relaxation exercises or as another adjunct to control panic and distress. The potential yet unconfirmed benefits of diaphragmatic breathing include increased tidal volume, reduced functional residual capacity, decreased oxygen cost of breathing, and presumably less dyspnea.[18] The application of abdominal or diaphragmatic breathing to directly relieve dyspnea has not been reported.

Again, the slowed respiratory rate and deeper tidal volume that may result from abdominal breathing may be the major reasons that patients report decreased breathlessness. Focusing on the efficient use of the diaphragm, especially during inspiration, may decrease the work of breathing, improve ventilation, and consequently reduce dyspnea. As with PLB, a slow, deep breathing pattern practiced in times of less shortness of breath also may help the patient feel more in control of breathing and decrease the anxiety that is associated with increasing dyspnea in acute or panic situations. Unfortunately, unless there is extensive practice, some patients may find the maneuver difficult to perform and may then revert to previously used patterns of breathing.

The patient should be taught to place his/her fingers below the sternum and sniff to locate the diaphragm. To detect movement of the diaphragm, one hand should be placed in the center of the stomach and another hand on the upper chest. The patient should inhale slowly through his/her nose and feel the abdomen push out under the hand as the diaphragm descends. Exhalation should be slow through pursed lips while the patient's hand pushes the abdomen inward and upward. Abdominal breathing should be practiced in different positions, including lying down and leaning forward. More detailed instructions of diaphragmatic breathing are outlined in Table 3. The patient also can be taught lower costal breathing that concentrates on expanding the lower lobes of the lungs. Patients should be encouraged to practice abdominal breathing with pursed lips at times other

Table 3. Diaphragmatic Breathing Directions

1. If you have a prescribed inhaled bronchodilator, take this medication before starting diaphragmatic breathing.
2. Lie flat or with your head tilted up.
3. Place one hand on your stomach just at the base or end of your breastbone—this hand will tell you when your diaphragm presses down against your abdomen, pushing your stomach out.
4. Place your other hand on your upper chest. Use this hand to tell you how much movement is occurring in your chest muscles.
5. Inhale slowly through your nose and allow your stomach to expand outward. Feel the pressure in your stomach; try to keep the upper chest from moving.
6. Then exhale slowly, remembering to use pursed-lips breathing.
7. Try to use only your diaphragm, pushing your abdomen out as much as you can.
8. Include rest periods.
9. Repeat this exercise until you feel comfortable using diaphragmatic and pursed-lips breathing together, lying down, then practice exercises sitting. Afterward, try exercises in a standing, leaning forward position.

than with acute episodes of dyspnea. Practice in both these combined techniques can help the patient to spontaneously use these strategies in situations of overwhelming dyspnea.

D. Graduated Levels of Dyspnea or "Desensitization"

One approach to "desensitizing" the anxious patient to exertional dyspnea is to encourage ambulation to the point that severe dyspnea occurs. The patient should be coached to use pursed-lips breathing techniques until comfort is regained.[19] If this technique is performed in a supportive environment with someone the patient trusts, the patient's fear of dyspnea may decrease while confidence is gained in the ability to control the symptom through his/her own actions. It is important to educate spouses or "significant others" to coach the patient so they can reinforce the breathing techniques during the time it takes for the patient to increase his/her skill and confidence.

E. Relaxation and Psychophysical Techniques

The close association between dyspnea and anxiety is well known.[20-22] If dyspnea is escalated and reinforced by anxiety, a strategy that decreases anxiety also may be expected to reduce the intensity and distress of dyspnea. In addition, Freedberg et al.[23] have suggested that relaxation can increase the ability of a patient to cope with a disease by helping the patient to exert greater control over associated symptoms.

Relaxation not only provides a response incompatible with anxiety and muscle tension in panic situations, but also helps the patient develop a behavioral self-care strategy that can be used on a daily basis to adapt to stress and to slow down the pace of life. Relaxation is based on the theory that individuals can focus attention on only one thing at a time. If the patient focuses on relaxation and/or decreasing muscle tension, his/her attention is diverted from anxiety associated with increasing shortness of breath. The practice of relaxation strengthens the patient's belief that, "I am in control." This strategy can help the patient exert some control during periods of increased breathlessness.[24]

Relaxation training has been evaluated more frequently in asthmatic patients[25-27] than those with chronic bronchitis or emphysema.[20] Various investigators have systematically studied progressive muscle relaxation techniques in pulmonary patients to determine the efficacy of relaxation on anxiety, respiratory rate, flow rates, and lung volumes, but not dyspnea.[20,23,25,28,29] In the laboratory setting, relaxation and biofeedback have been shown to reduce respiratory rate, total respiratory resistance, and tidal volume in selected patients.[29,30]

There are a variety of different techniques that patients can be taught to help them relax during exacerbations of severe dyspnea and/or panic, as well as to decrease stress in daily life. Progressive muscle relaxation[31] and the Jacobsonian relaxation method[32] are two widely used techniques. Common components of most relaxation techniques include the following:

1. a quiet environment
2. a comfortable position
3. loose, non-restrictive clothing
4. adoption of a passive attitude
5. some type of word or imagery repeated or thought of in a systematic fashion
6. slow abdominal breathing with deep inhalation and slow exhalation through pursed lips
7. systematic tensing or relaxing every part of the body including

feet, arms, legs, chest, etc., concentrating on each muscle as
the tension or relaxation is prolonged

It is important to explain to patients that there are many different
approaches for relaxation and that the health-care provider will work
closely with the patient to find the most suitable techniques. Live
instructions, demonstration, and practice have been found to produce
more positive outcomes. Therefore, it is preferable for an instructor to
be present to give feedback and encouragement whenever possible.
Taped instructions can be used in the home for practice and to enhance
the patient's independence and self-esteem. Individualized tape recordings that describe specific solutions can be used to coach someone
though relaxation techniques during the panic of dyspnea in the
home.[33]

Practice is essential in order for the patient to become skillful
enough to use relaxation in acute panic situations. Relaxation works
well for some patients but not for others. Some patients can use
relaxation daily to decrease their stress, while others can use relaxation only for panic episodes. However, additional research is needed
to determine whether relaxation techniques significantly decrease
dyspnea. Relaxation appears to decrease anxiety, and this may be the
mechanism by which it relieves dyspnea for some patients.

Other psychophysiological techniques that are used clinically for
helping dyspnea include visual imagery, biofeedback, and meditation.[20,29,34] These strategies need to be individualized. It is probably
most important to encourage the patient to practice some type of
relaxation every day in order to prepare for severe dyspneic situations.

F. Activity Modification and Energy Conservation

Some of the most difficult tasks for patients with shortness of
breath are to learn to pace their activities, to slow down, and to
conserve energy. Patients need help and support in making major
lifestyle changes as shortness of breath begins to affect their activity
tolerance. The patient can be helped to modify or substitute activities
that are pleasurable but require less effort. For example, if gardening
is too difficult, caring for house plants may be just as much fun.
Hobbies such as playing cards can be suggested for less strenuous
activity to replace the weekly golf game. The health-care provider

needs to work with the patient to choose alternative pleasurable activities within his/her usual lifestyle and social environment. Patients need help with planning in advance for almost any activity. Vacations and trips should be organized early to allow time to anticipate the availability of oxygen, the altitude, the amount of energy the trip will require, and the scheduling of rest periods. Daily walks, restaurant lunches, and activities need to be planned ahead of time to anticipate "breathing stations," exact activities for the day, week, and month, and energy that will have to be used each day. Most practitioners suggest a "daily outline," dividing the day into morning, afternoon, late afternoon, and early evening. After deciding what daily tasks must be done, they can be divided across the day, leaving time for scheduled rests and leisure or pleasurable activities. Patients should be taught to make rest periods a high priority, diligently scheduling them before and after any activity that increases shortness of breath. If there is a period of the day when the patient feels best, he/she should set aside that time for the most demanding activities.

Patients should be instructed that there is a crucial balance between pacing or resting and appropriate exercise. Graduated exercise and activity to stay physically conditioned and use oxygen efficiently has to be stressed while at the same time emphasizing the needs for a slower pace. Teaching should include contrasting the energy used for tasks that are unnecessary with energy that is used for leisure activities and daily exercises that will enhance the efficiency of the muscles and the body.

Patients should be given specific recommendations for completing activities of daily living such as grooming, bathing, showering, and dressing. Major instructions are outlined in Table 4. It is important to review steps in self-care with the patient so that management can be individualized for the patient's ability, daily routine, and home environment.

To decrease dyspnea with activities of daily living, occupational therapists often teach patients how to perform daily tasks more efficiently with less energy expenditure. Avoiding unnecessary motions includes minimizing steps in any task, avoiding overreaching and bending by arranging equipment closely, using good posture and body mechanics, using good breathing techniques in performing any task, and sitting when possible. Setting up proper working conditions includes working at proper work height, avoiding clutter in work

---

Table 4. Energy Conservation in Grooming and Dressing

Grooming

- Sit when possible for brushing teeth, makeup, etc.
- Avoid aerosols or strongly scented perfumes that increase shortness of breath.
- Consider short hair cuts; wash hair in shower.
- Support yourself with elbows if you possibly can to decrease shortness of breath.

Bathing and Showering

- Use a chair or stool in the shower or tub.
- Sit to bathe, dry, dress, and undress.
- Consider using a terry cloth bathrobe to pat self dry.
- Use lukewarm water that reduces steam and does not increase shortness of breath.
- Use oxygen in shower or bath if it decreases shortness of breath.
- Take rest periods.
- Non-skid strips and grab bars help you keep balance.
- Use a shower hose extension to control direction of water and avoid standing to rinse.
- Keep soap handy with soap-rope or suction cap.

Dressing

- Have a dressing area where all clothes can be reached easily.
- Sit on edge of bed or chair to dress.
- Dress the lower body first and upper body last.
- Decrease shortness of breath by putting underwear and pants on at the same time.
- Decrease bending by crossing one leg over the other while sitting to put on socks, trousers, and shoes.
- Use pursed-lips breathing during all activities.
- Use slip-on shoes and long-handled shoehorn.

---

area, breaking the job down into steps, and streamlining by eliminating all unnecessary details and combining motions and activities.

There are extensive published lists of recommendations to help patients conserve energy and minimize shortness of breath during homemaking chores, such as meal preparation, washing/ironing, and cleaning.[35-37] The American Lung Association (ALA) and local organizations offer a variety of pamphlets on energy conservation for patients. Important instructions available to patients to help alleviate their shortness of breath during activities of daily living are summarized in Table 5.

Table 5. Energy Conservation in Homemaking

Cooking/Meal Preparation

* Plan meals in advance. Allow yourself plenty of time to prepare meals so that you do not feel rushed. Having extra time will allow for rest periods, if needed.

* Gather all necessary food and utensils from cupboards and refrigerator. Use breathing pattern for reaching up into cupboard, inhaling when raising arms and exhaling as you bring arms down. Use breathing pattern for stooping to lower cupboards (exhale when stooping). Break this activity into steps if necessary. Try to work with arms close to body; do not overextend yourself if it is not necessary.

* After all necessary items have been placed on counter or cart, transfer them to work area where you can sit (either at a table or at a counter with a high kitchen stool). If items must be transferred to another area, try to make only one trip. It is advisable to use a rolling tea cart for this.

* Set the table in the same manner for gathering; if table area is small enough, stay in one position to set table. If reaching across table causes difficulty, use reaching pattern (inhale when extending arms, exhale on return); if setting a large table, set one side at a time. Consider eating meals in the kitchen or breakfast room.

* Use an electric mixer, if one is available, rather than mixing by hand.

* Eliminate unnecessary steps and processes:
  a. let dishes drain dry, sit on a high stool when washing dishes.
  b. use paper dinner napkins instead of linen ones.
  c. use placemats instead of tablecloths.
  d. soak pots in hot water and detergent to eliminate vigorous scouring.

* If possible, use counter to slide heavy pots and other articles to avoid unnecessary carrying. If you must carry objects, use both hands and keep object close to body.

* Try to cut down in any way possible to eliminate unnecessary steps and work. Use prepared, frozen, or prepackaged foods and one-dish casseroles. Cut down on dishes by using heat-resistant cookware that allows heating and serving in the same dish.

* Prepare extra portions of food and freeze the excess for future use.

Cleaning

* For large cleaning, allow entire day as this is a big job to tackle.

* Clean one room at a time and do not allow yourself to be distracted by another room that also needs cleaning. It can wait. If cleaning entire house would be too fatiguing, clean one room a day to spread out the job.

(continued)

Table 5. *Continued*

- To wash floors, use a long-handled dustpan and sponge mop. Use tongs to pick up objects from the floor. Using breathing pattern, inhale as you push mop away from you, exhale as you pull it towards you. Vacuum using the same pattern with pursed-lips breathing.

- Dusting may cause difficulty as the dust itself may be an irritant. Some dusting may be done while sitting. Do not use spray wax as this may be an irritant also. Instead, use a cream or paste wax for polishing furniture. Work in a pattern around the room.

- Windows can be washed using a breathing pattern to reach. Again, do not use spray cleaner if it can be helped; water and vinegar work just as well.

- When other objects must be removed from the room being cleaned, put them in a basket or on a rolling tea cart for later distribution. Do not run from one room to another while trying to clean.

- If furniture must be moved, have someone else move it for you.

- Cleaning out cupboards also can be done using a systemized technique. Use a pattern of inhaling as you reach and exhaling as object is brought down, and vice versa. Again, avoid spray cleaners.

- Use aluminum foil and oven bags where possible to eliminate unnecessary scrubbing. If this is not always possible, soak pan immediately after use for easier cleaning or use vegetable spray.

- To clean bathtub, sit beside tub or on tub edge. Use long-handled brush or sponge to avoid reaching or bending.

- Dish washing should be done while sitting on a high kitchen stool, opening cupboard beneath to allow for leg room. Scalding dishes and allowing them to air dry will eliminate drying. Allow rest before returning dishes to cupboards.

- Organize your home to your advantage, keeping items in the most convenient places and always returning them there.

Bedmaking
- Make one side of the bed at a time. When changing bed linen, put bottom sheet, top sheet, blanket, and spread on, then tuck in bottom sheet at both ends. Continue making bed on that side as usual.

- When shaking out bed linen, use breathing pattern of inhaling as you raise your arms, exhaling as you bring linen onto bed. When smoothing bed clothes, if reach is significant, use breathing pattern again of inhaling as you extend and exhaling as you pull towards your body.

- If this task is a difficult one for you, stooping can eliminate some unnecessary bending. If necessary, this can be done sitting for at least part of the activities.

Table 5. *Continued*

- Beds on casters or rollers are easier to move, but should have locks.
- Beds are easier to make if away from the walls (or only head against walls).
- An electric blanket keeps in body heat, is light in weight, and is less for the body to support all night.

Washing/Ironing
- When possible, have family members bring clothes to laundry room.
- If possible, use a rolling laundry cart and sort clothes on a table (never on the floor).
- If you have to hand wash, sit if at all possible. Wash in pan at proper height. Try soaking clothes rather than scrubbing.
- If laundry facilities are in the basement, have a chair in the laundry area if you do not feel you can make frequent trips up and down the stairs.
- Put front-loading washer on blocks to raise opening and thus eliminate the necessity of bending.
- Send heavy clothes, i.e., bedspreads, curtains, rugs, to commercial laundry. Use reaching tongs to remove articles. Sit to fold laundry.
- Do not iron, just fold, sheets, towels, and underwear. Buy permanent press or easy care articles.
- Always sit to iron with board at lap level. Again, when distributing ironed and/or dried clothing, make one trip in a sequenced manner.
- Slide iron, do not lift it or set it on end. Place it on an asbestos pad while adjusting clothes on board.

Adapted from Wilson B. *Pacing and Energy Conservation in Pulmonary Rehabilitation.* Winnipeg, Manitoba, Occupational Therapy Department, General Hospital of Port Arthur, 1987, with permission.

G. Strategies for Decreasing Dyspnea during Sexual Activity

When patients are able to confide in a health professional in whom they have developed trust, they frequently complain of dyspnea during sexual activity. As with other activities, patients can be taught strategies to decrease energy expenditure and, therefore, dyspnea. Suggestions include use of a rest period and inhaled bronchodilators before sexual relations, "passive" positions, use of supplemental oxygen, appropriate timing of sexual relations before meals and after resting, and avoiding positions that require supporting body weight or that increase pressure on the chest. Patients who still experience intense dyspnea during intercourse can be reminded of other expressions of love, including holding, embracing, or caressing.[38]

H. Eating and Meal Preparation

People who are short of breath often become anorexic because eating contributes to shortness of breath. Individual patients avoid eating to minimize episodes of increasing dyspnea. Reasons for dyspnea during eating are unknown, but the increased energy required for chewing and arm movements, the reduction in airflow while swallowing, and oxygen desaturation are proposed mechanisms.[39] Self-care strategies to decrease dyspnea during eating include the following:

1. preparing meals in advance
2. assuming a body position that makes breathing easier and using pursed-lips breathing
3. preparing small meals and food that is easy to chew
4. using oxygen during meals
5. avoiding a high carbohydrate diet and gas-producing foods

Patients who experience chronic dyspnea often are malnourished and have been unable to eat adequate amounts for long periods of time. However, there is another group of patients who may have gained weight. Patients who have gained weight due to prolonged corticosteroid use and/or lack of activity may experience increased dyspnea from abdominal "loading." These patients should be encouraged to lose weight by active meal planning, a nutritious diet, constant encouragement at each visit to lose weight, and referral to a weight loss group or program. When patients are told that weight gain can increase their dyspnea, they may be more motivated to adhere to dietary restrictions and weight loss programs.

I. Seeking Social Support

Social support has been found to buffer stress in chronic diseases and stressful situations.[40] Janson-Bjerklie et al.[41] reported that the level of dyspnea experienced by patients with pulmonary disease was related to the number of persons in the social support network and the frequency of contact with others. The amount of material aid, affirmation, and affection were also positively related to the intensity of dyspnea. Although some patients with severe dyspnea had become socially isolated, many others had developed extensive networks and resources that provided high levels of social support.[41]

In our clinical practice, we have observed that when patients are able to increase both the number of people in their social network and their use of community resources, the distress of their dyspnea seems to diminish. Support group meetings, such as ALA Better Breathers Clubs, allow time for patients to share common distressful experiences and strategies they have used to alleviate their dyspnea. Sharing common feelings and problems about living with shortness of breath helps people find alternative strategies to cope with the symptom. Ashikaga and colleagues[42] found that patients with COPD increased their use of self-help skills at home after a group workshop. Group approval, encouragement, and support promoted attitudinal changes that increased confidence and motivation. Support, warmth, enthusiasm, and genuine caring, whether from a health-care provider or from people who are suffering from the same symptom, are important factors in allaying a patient's anxiety and decreasing dyspnea.[43] Support groups give a patient the opportunity to see that he/she is not alone and that others have accomplished adaptive outcomes to the same chronic problem.[44] Family members also need support and should be included in group sessions.

Many patients who have been independent and productive members of a family and community find themselves dependent on family and friends. Patients need assistance in learning to take on another role and accept help from these same people. Active support from family or friends can be a buffer and can change a person's negative interpretation of a stressful event, such as dyspnea, to a positive one.[44] Many patients with dyspnea experience a loss of network, either because they have to leave their lifelong job or they cannot continue the activity that brought them in contact with a usual group of friends. Health-care professionals need to be aware of the patient's need for a certain level of support and should intervene either by focusing on changing the informal network and/or by providing formal support resources to supplement the attention and help provided by family and friends.

Patients should be taught to tell "significant others" and family members how they can specifically help and how to look for behaviors and signs that indicate changes in the level of dyspnea. People with COPD have identified behaviors, including panting, wheezing, coughing, and being very quiet and withdrawn, that are outward manifestations of increasing dyspnea that can be observed by others.[41]

J. Increasing Knowledge and Education

Although knowledge itself has not been shown to decrease dyspnea or increase compliance with self-care strategies, preparatory information about anticipated sensations has been shown to decrease anxiety and increase the patient's perception of control over impending distress.[45] Knowledge of risk factors or triggers of episodes of dyspnea enables the patient to manipulate environmental and personal situations either by staying away from the precipitant, taking preparatory medications, relaxing, or using breathing strategies to minimize the distress of the event. Triggers that most often increase dyspnea should be discussed with the patient. This discussion should allow the patients to identify those factors that in the past have brought on or intensified their dyspneic episodes. Patients should be taught principles of self-care to be used for both acute and chronic dyspnea as described in Tables 6 and 7, respectively.

Table 6. Tips for Coping with Acute Episodes of Dyspnea

1. Assess severity of the episode by rating how short of breath you feel on a scale of 1 to 10.
2. Monitor changes in your body that alert you to increased shortness of breath. Call health-care provider if shortness of breath changes in frequency or intensity. If you have asthma, measure peak flow rate with a peak flow meter. If the value is lower than your baseline, use a metered-dose inhaler with sustained inspiration and breath-holding. Take a second puff and then measure peak flow rate again. Tell your health-care provider the values you have recorded when you call.
3. Use all the techniques you have learned to decrease your shortness of breath: pursed-lip breathing, relaxation, abdominal breathing, position, fluids, fans, and medication, including those delivered by nebulizer. Simple relaxation or meditation strategies may relax you and permit slower, deeper breathing, thus allowing a sense of control over breathing.
4. Evaluate your response to the strategies and medications you have tried. If symptoms have not markedly improved, proceed to the clinic, doctor's office, or emergency room without delay.

Table 7. Tips for Coping with Chronic Dyspnea

1. Know your own pattern of episodes. Monitor your shortness of breath. Know what brings your attacks on or makes them worse. Make it predictable! Evaluate severity of episodes by rating how short of breath you feel on a scale of 1 to 10. Monitor signs of infection such as tightness, changes in sputum, fatigue, and increased cough; start medication, oxygen, etc., as necessary.
2. If you have asthma, measure peak flow at least daily in the early morning upon arising, before medications. Know your normal baseline peak flow. Measure twice daily before medications in the early morning and at bedtime, if possible. If peak flow drops in the A.M. to 50% of the P.M. value or 50% of previous known value for 2 days, seek help from health-care provider. Keep a record of your peak flow. When you have an altered pattern, know what your baseline is and how far you have deviated from your normal baseline.
3. Identify and prioritize strategies that work for you to reduce the intensity and distress of your symptoms. Use any techniques that decrease your shortness of breath in the order that works best for you. Try to exercise every day and "move through" graduated levels of shortness of breath so you can tolerate more shortness of breath.
4. Have a crisis plan. Know what you will do in the event of a severe episode that does not get better with medications that you carry with you. Know how to get to medical help quickly. Have a partner or friend that you can call for help to get to the emergency room or the clinic quickly.
5. Plan ahead. Before going into a new situation, think of what you will do if you become short of breath. Keep resources and medications handy. Don't get caught without your medicine and other resources that help you get through a situation. Anticipate activities, plan far ahead so you can conserve energy and make arrangements, and determine "breathing stations."
6. Get the information and the data that you need to cope with shortness of breath by forming a partnership in self-management with your health-care provider. Prepare a list of questions you want answered before you go to your clinic appointments. Ask for resources and help, including phone numbers to use when you need advice and support. Ask your health-care provider what the medications that are ordered are supposed to do for you and what you can reasonably expect. Teach other people, including physicians, nurses, and family, the strategies that you have learned so they can help you use them during acute shortness of breath.

Strategies that patients have identified in the past to help minimize dyspnea can be combined with those that other patients have found to be successful. A larger repertoire of strategies to minimize dyspnea may, in fact, decrease the frequency and intensity of episodes. The belief of patients that they have behavioral strategies to cope with a symptom has been found to decrease the distress of that symptom.[9]

K. Symptom Monitoring

Daily monitoring of the intensity and frequency of the symptom can help patients become aware of the fluctuations in breathlessness with daily activities, emotional changes, or environmental patterns. Having a baseline and daily log of the trajectory of the symptoms may improve the patient's awareness of those strategies that either aggravate or alleviate dyspnea and may increase the perception of control over the symptom. In this way, patients may see changes in scores of symptom intensity as they begin a certain treatment or stop smoking. Self-monitoring can also include physiological information, such as peak expiratory flow rate (PF), especially for those who have asthma. The peak flow meter provides feedback of information about the degree of airflow limitation. Patients with asthma can be taught to use PF measurements to adjust medication dosage and frequency, alter self-management practices, and initiate contact with the health-care provider. In other disease conditions, self-monitoring has been reported to increase the patient's understanding of his/her disease[46] and to boost an individual's confidence.[47] The patient's perception of control appears to increase as he/she monitors dyspnea over time.

L. Contracting for Goals

Therapeutic goals can be written in a formal contract in order to promote mutual understanding and to clarify the responsibilities of the health-care provider, the patient, and family members. Contracts usually are designed to specify behavior-consequence relationships and involve two people in monitoring, reminding, and participating in the regimen and/or giving reinforcement.[6] Setting goals with a patient can be used to involve the patient in decision making about what strategies are appropriate and successful for his/her individual lifestyle and may increase adherence with the agreed upon regimen for alleviating dyspnea.[48] Goals that are attainable can serve as benchmarks to evaluate progress in decreasing the distress of the symptom.

In one study, patients with chronic bronchitis and emphysema who participated in a rehabilitation program were encouraged to set their own goals, prioritize problems, and try the therapy that worked best. These patients experienced a significant decrease in the frequency of symptoms.[49]

M. Attitudes and Life Change

Many people with chronic lung disease state that their lives have been changed dramatically by altering either their attitudes toward themselves and their disease or by altering their lifestyle. Changing one's attitude toward disease usually means adopting the perception of self as a healthy person instead of a sick person. Those with chronic pulmonary disease who become disabled by distressful symptoms such as dyspnea tend to become more physically and socially limited and see themselves as ill.

An exercise program is one of the most powerful generators of change in attitude toward life and symptom management (see Chapter 8). A carefully planned exercise program lets patients progress in a step-wise fashion to higher levels of tolerance while competence and self-esteem grow. A successful program can lead to a new and more positive outlook where "anything is possible." Those who have accomplished such a change describe an increased sense of control and mastery, empowerment, and positive self-image. They begin to see themselves as healthy, not sick. These changes in attitude often are accompanied by decreased distress and a greater tolerance of dyspnea.

N. Self-Management of Medication Regimen

Management of dyspnea in the face of severe episodic symptoms may require the patient to learn to manipulate complex medication regimens. Altering the dose or frequency of the medication or adding a new drug may be necessary without contact with the health-care provider. Patients can learn to do this with support from the physician and with access to direct feedback information, such as PF or visual analogue scale measurements (see Chapter 3), of symptom intensity. Inhaled bronchodilators may be used more frequently or the number of puffs may be increased. When a more severe episode of bronchoconstriction develops over a period of 1 to 2 days, the patient with adequate information and support may be able to start corticosteroid therapy and then contact the physician for confirmation. Such manipulation of a complex therapeutic regimen takes a great deal of skill and knowledge on the part of the patient and shared trust between physician and patient.

O. Self-Care Strategies Presented in Pulmonary Rehabilitation Programs

Pulmonary rehabilitation programs frequently enable patients to experience a reduction in respiratory symptoms and to increase their ability to carry out activities of daily living.[50,51] However, it is difficult to determine the true effect of the multiple components of pulmonary rehabilitation programs on the intensity and frequency of dyspnea.

Although different instruments and time periods were used, selected studies have shown that pulmonary rehabilitation programs may have a positive effect on the symptom of dyspnea.[52–57] Fishman and Petty[52] compared the clinical status of 30 COPD patients upon entry into a comprehensive care program and 1 year later. Patients were questioned whether their "lung illness caused them breathing difficulty" at the present time compared to the previous year. "Breathing difficulty" decreased, although not significantly, and the "difficulty" compared with the previous year was rated significantly less by these patients. The change consisted of a stabilization of symptoms during the first year of the program compared to a pattern of symptom deterioration during the previous year.

Moser and colleagues[53] evaluated 42 COPD patients as part of a 6-week comprehensive rehabilitation program that included patient education, group psychotherapy, and individualized programs of chest physiotherapy and exercise. They found that 16 of the 29 patients in dyspnea classes 2 to 5 improved 1 class or more (on a scale with ratings of absent, small degree, moderate, severe, or intolerable dyspnea) during a range of activities.[53]

In a retrospective study of 75 COPD patients who had participated in a 2-week pulmonary rehabilitation program, Bebout and colleagues[54] found that the dyspnea classification improved in 53% of the patients, did not change in 19%, and became worse in 28%. The dyspnea classification was modified from a 5-point grading scale related to activity.[55] Two additional studies suggest that outpatient programs improve dyspnea in symptomatic patients.[56,57]

At the present time, it is unknown which of the individual components of these programs modulates dyspnea. Coping strategies emphasized in most rehabilitation programs include education, exercise, psychological support, attention, breathing retraining, and social interaction. Controlled clinical trials are needed to examine the effect of these individual components on the intensity and distress of dyspnea.

P. Formal Psychotherapy

Learning strategies to decrease dyspnea that give the patient control of the anxiety/dyspnea cycle often help to decrease the frequency of anxiety or depression. However, if depression and/or anxiety appear to be major contributors to increasing intensity or frequency of shortness of breath, formal sessions with a psychiatrist or psychologist may help these disturbances. The use of anxiolytic and antidepressant medications has been reviewed elsewhere[43,58] (see Chapter 8). To insure an appropriate medication regimen, it is important to distinguish between psychiatric disease and mood disturbances that are expected reactions to chronic illness. Formal psychotherapy has been reported to be a successful part of pulmonary rehabilitation.[59] However, the effect of psychotherapy on dyspnea remains unknown.

Q. Strategies Reported by Patients with Dyspnea

The self-care and coping strategies actually used by COPD patients have been characterized through descriptive research. Fagerhaugh[60] and Barstow[61] each categorized behaviors used by emphysema patients to manage activities of daily living and social relationships. Barstow[61] described general strategies such as postponing, prioritizing, and careful advanced planning to minimize energy expenditure and reduce breathlessness. A significant person in the household (social support), financial well-being, possession of a car, and an efficacious medical regimen were important factors that promoted adjustment. Fagerhaugh[60] identified money, time, energy, "breathing stations," and "mobility assistants" as important determinants of successful coping. Other major adaptive strategies included recording of time, managing the illness trajectory, normalizing, management of regimens, and controlling the symptom.

Chalmers[62] described 3 categories of coping strategies used by 30 patients with COPD. Behavioral strategies or actions to deal with the effects of the disease included taking medications, making environmental alterations, and avoiding precipitants. Cognitive strategies included focusing on the positive aspects of life, normalization or minimization, pacing activities, reminiscing and reflection, and problem solving. Expressive strategies were expressions of emotions that helped the patient adjust to the disease.

Carrieri and Janson-Bjerklie[11] interviewed 68 individuals who experienced dyspnea as a result of obstructive, restrictive, or pulmonary vascular disease. Irrespective of the disease category, all subjects found ways to cope with their dyspnea. These patients used and taught themselves various types of self-care strategies for long-term adaptive changes and coping strategies for acute new situations. Successful strategies were more problem-focused than emotion-focused. Asthmatic patients developed the greatest number of coping strategies. Of note, the strategies commonly taught to patients experiencing dyspnea were not always useful for patients with restrictive and vascular disease. The adaptive strategies and changes in lifestyle used by the emphysema-bronchitis group were similar to those reported by others. In general, these subjects made the same types of changes in activities of daily living by modifying and pacing their daily activity. They used advanced planning of activities, resting places, complex medication regimens, and avoidance of precipitating situations in order to cope with shortness of breath. Even very specific strategies for reducing acute dyspnea were described, such as turning on a fan or sitting by an open window allowing cool air to blow directly on the face. The use of cool air generated by fans to reduce dyspnea has been tested with a sample of normal subjects.[63] Although breathless patients with pulmonary vascular disease who required continuous oxygen had not been taught strategies for coping, these patients changed their lifestyle radically by slowing their pace and severely restricting activities.[11]

Most importantly, there were differences in the number and type of strategies used by patients across different disease categories. The type and frequency of strategies were determined by the characteristics of the symptom. The strategies that patients adopt can change with the frequency, periodicity, and intensity of dyspnea. Patients have the ability to develop their own individual strategies to cope with dyspnea, and these strategies should be incorporated into the plan of care.

V. Summary

Coping with the distressful symptom of dyspnea is an ongoing and complex process that involves education, skill attainment, and constant adjustment. To promote coping with dyspnea, approaches and strategies must be individualized to specific life situations. Whether breathing techniques, relaxation, or social support strategies are most effective depends on the specific situation that aggravates dyspnea. The goal is to decrease the frequency and intensity of dyspnea; when that is not possible, the effort should be directed to minimize the distress that each patient experiences.

References

1. Dudley DL, Glaser EM, Jorgenson BN, et al. Psychosocial concomitants to rehabilitation in chronic obstructive pulmonary disease. I. Pyschosocial and psychological considerations. Chest 1980; 77:413-420.
2. Dudley DL, Glaser EM, Jorgenson BN, et al. Psychosocial concomitants to rehabilitation in chronic obstructive pulmonary disease. II. Psychosocial treatment. Chest 1980; 77:544-551.
3. Strauss AL, Corbin J, Fagerhaugh S, et al. Chronic Illness and the Quality of Life, 2nd Edition. St. Louis, C.V. Mosby Co., 1984.
4. Lazarus RS, Folkman S. Stress, Appraisal and Coping. New York, Springer Publishing Co., 1984.
5. Folkman S, Lazarus RS. Coping as a mediator of emotion. J Pers Soc Psychol 1988; 54:466-475.
6. Holroyd KA, Creer TL. Self-Management of Chronic Disease: Handbook of Clinical Interventions and Research. Orlando, Academic Press Inc., 1986.
7. Carrieri VK, Janson-Bjerklie S, Jacobs S. The sensation of dyspnea. A review. Heart Lung 1984; 13:436-447.
8. Lazarus RS, Folkman S. Coping and adaptation. In: Gentry WD (ed). The Handbook of Behavioral Medicine. New York, W.D.Guilford, 1984; 282-325.
9. Thompson SC. Will it hurt less if I can control it? A complex answer to a simple question. Psychol Bull 1981; 90:89-101.

10. Folkman S, Lazarus RS. If it changes it must be a process: study of emotion and coping during three states of college examination. J Pers Soc Psychol 1985; 48:150-170.
11. Carrieri VK, Janson-Bjerklie S. Strategies patients use to manage the sensation of dyspnea. West J Nurs Res 1986; 8:284-305.
12. Shekleton M. Coping with chronic respiratory difficulty. Nurs Clin North Am 1987; 22:569-581.
13. Sharp JT, Drutz WS, Moisan T, et al. Postural relief of dyspnea in severe chronic obstructive pulmonary disease. Am Rev Respir Dis 1980; 122: 201-213.
14. Lareau S, Larson JL. Ineffective breathing pattern related to airflow limitation. Nurs Clin North Am 1987; 22:179-191.
15. Mueller RE, Petty TL, Filley GF. Ventilation and arterial blood gas changes induced by pursed lips breathing. J Appl Physiol 1970; 28:784-789.
16. Thoman RL, Stoker GL, Ross JC. The efficacy of pursed lips breathing in patients with chronic obstructive pulmonary disease. Am Rev Respir Dis 1966; 93:100-106.
17. Tiep BL, Burns M, Kao D. Pursed-lips breathing training using ear oximetry. Chest 1986; 90:218-221.
18. Hodgkin JE, Petty TL. Chronic Obstructive Pulmonary Disease: Current Concepts. Philadelphia, W.B. Saunders Co., 1987.
19. Agle DP, Baum GL, Chester EH, et al. Multidiscipline treatment of chronic pulmonary insufficiency. I. Psychologic aspects of rehabilitation. Psychosom Med 1973; 35:41-49.
20. Renfroe KL. Effect of progressive relaxation on dyspnea and state anxiety in patients with chronic obstructive pulmonary disease. Heart Lung 1988; 17:408-413.
21. Rosser R, Denford J, Heslop A, et al. Breathlessness and psychiatric morbidity in chronic bronchitis and emphysema: a study of psychotherapeutic management. Psychol Med 1983; 13:93-110.
22. Gift A, Plaut M, Jacox A. Psychologic and physiologic factors related to dyspnea in subjects with chronic obstructive pulmonary disease. Heart Lung 1986; 15:595-601.
23. Freedberg PD, Hoffman LA, Light WC, et al. Effect of progressive muscle relaxation on the objective symptoms and subjective responses associated with asthma. Heart Lung 1987; 16:24-30.
24. Turk DC, Holzman AD, Kerns RD. Chronic pain. In: Holroyd KA, Creer TL (eds). Self-Management of Chronic Disease. Florida, Academic Press, 1986; 441-472.
25. Alexander A, Miklich D, Hershkoff H. The immediate effects of systematic relaxation training on peak expiratory flow rates in asthmatic children. Psychosom Med 1972; 24:388-394.
26. Philipp R, Wilde G, Day J. Suggestion and relaxation in asthmatics. J Psychosom Res 1972; 16:193-204.
27. Hock R, Rodgers C, Reddi C, et al. Medico-psychological interventions in male asthmatic children. Psychosom Med 1978; 40:210-215.

28. Acosta F. Biofeedback and progressive relaxation in weaning the anxious patient from the ventilator: a brief report. Heart Lung 1988; 17:299-301.
29. Sitzman J, Kamiya J, Johnston J. Biofeedback training for reduced respiratory rate in chronic obstructive pulmonary disease: a preliminary study. Nurs Res 1983; 32:218-223.
30. Janson-Bjerklie S, Clarke E. The effects of biofeedback training on bronchial diameter in asthma. Heart Lung 1982; 11:200.
31. Benson H. The Relaxation Response. New York, Morrow Co., 1975.
32. Bernstein DA, Borkovec TD. Progressive relaxation training. A manual for the helping professions. Champaign, Illinois, Research Press, 1973.
33. Horsman J. Using tape recordings to overcome panic during dyspnea. Respir Care 1978; 23:767-768.
34. Vines SW. The therapeutics of guided imagery. Holistic Nurs Prac 1988; 2:34-44.
35. Hopp JW, Hodgkin JE, Maddox-Perez SE, et al. Living with Lung Disease: A Patient Handbook. Loma Linda, California, Loma Linda University, 1985.
36. St. Helena Hospital and Health Center. Pulmonary Rehabilitation Patient Education Manual, 1987.
37. Wilson B. Pacing and Energy Conservation in Pulmonary Rehabilitation. Winnipeg, Manitoba, Occupational Therapy Department Rehabilitation Center, General Hospital of Port Arthur, 1987.
38. Sexton DL. Chronic Obstructive Pulmonary Disease: Care of the Child and Adult. St. Louis, C.V. Mosby Co., 1981.
39. Neagley SR, Zwillich CW. The influence of gastric filling and caloric consumption on the sensation of dyspnea in COPD (abstract). Am Rev Respir Dis 1986; 133(suppl): A163.
40. Cobb S. Social support as a moderator of life stress. Psychosom Med 1976; 38:300-314.
41. Janson-Bjerklie S, Carrieri VK, Hudes M. The sensations of pulmonary dyspnea. Nurs Res 1986; 35:154-159.
42. Ashikaga T, Vacek PM, Lewis SO. Evaluation of a community-based education program for individuals with chronic obstructive pulmonary disease. J Rehabil 1980; 46:23-27.
43. Sandhu HS. Psychosocial issues in chronic obstructive pulmonary disease. Clin Chest Med 1986; 7:629-642.
44. Burkhardt CS. Coping strategies of the chronically ill. Nurs Clin North Am 1987; 22:543-550.
45. Johnson JE. The effects of accurate expectations about sensations on the sensory and distress components of pain. J Pers Soc Psychol 1973; 27:261-275.
46. Walford S, Zale EAM, Allison SP, et al. Self-monitoring of blood-glucose. Improvement of diabetic control. Lancet 1978; i:732-735.
47. Worth R, Hoome PD, Johnston DG, et al. Intensive attention improves glycaemic control in insulin-dependent diabetes without further advantage from home blood glucose monitoring: results of a controlled trial. Br Med J 1982; 285:1233-1240.

48. Herje PA. Hows and whys of patient contracting. Nurse Educator 1980; 5:30-34.
49. Perry JA. Effectiveness of teaching in the rehabilitation of patients with chronic bronchitis and emphysema. Nurs Res 1981; 30:219-222.
50. Hodgkin JE, Asmus RM, Conners GA. Pulmonary rehabilitation: designing a program that works. J Respir Dis 1987; 8:55-68.
51. Ries AL. Pulmonary rehabilitation. In: Fishman AP (ed). Pulmonary Diseases and Disorders, Vol. 2, 2nd Edition. New York, McGraw-Hill Book Co., 1982.
52. Fishman DB, Petty TL. Physical, symptomatic and psychological improvement in patients receiving comprehensive care for chronic airway obstruction. J Chronic Dis 1971; 24:775-785.
53. Moser KN, Bokinsky GE, Savage RT, et al. Results of a comprehensive rehabilitation program. Arch Intern Med 1980; 140:1596-1601.
54. Bebout DE, Hodgkin JE, Zorn EG, et al. Clinical and physiological outcomes of a university-hospital pulmonary rehabilitation program. Respir Care 1983; 28:1468-1473.
55. Kimbel P, Kaplan AS, Alkalay I, et al. An in-hospital program for rehabilitation of patients with chronic obstructive pulmonary disease. Chest 1971; 60:65-105.
56. Mal RW, Medeiros M. Objective evaluation of results of a pulmonary rehabilitation program in a community hospital. Chest 1988; 94:1156-1160.
57. Atkins CJ, Kaplan RM, Timms RM, et al. Behavioral exercise programs in the management of chronic obstructive pulmonary disease. J Consult Clin Psychol 1984; 52:591-603.
58. Rosser R, Guz A. Psychological approaches to breathlessness and its treatment. J Psychosom Res 1981; 25:439-447.
59. Agle DP, Baum GL, Chester EH, et al. Multidiscipline treatment of chronic pulmonary insufficiency. I. Psychologic aspects of rehabilitation. Psychosom Med 1973; 35:41-49.
60. Fagerhaugh SY. Getting around with emphysema. Am J Nurs 1973; 72: 94-100.
61. Barstow R. Coping with emphysema. Nurs Clin North Am 1974; 9:137-145.
62. Chalmers KT. A closer look at how people cope with chronic airflow obstruction. Can Nurse 1984; 80:35-38.
63. Schwartzstein RM, Lahive K, Pope A, et al. Cold facial stimulation reduces breathlessness induced in normal subjects. Am Rev Respir Dis 1987; 136:58-61.

Chapter 8

Therapeutic Strategies

Donald A. Mahler

I. Introduction

What are the goals of therapy for chronic respiratory disease?
To answer this question, it is important to consider the natural

From *Dyspnea*, edited by Donald A. Mahler, M.D., © 1990, Futura Publishing
Company, Inc., Mount Kisco, NY.

history and mortality of the particular chronic respiratory disorder. The following discussion focuses on these two issues in chronic obstructive pulmonary disease (COPD), the most frequent respiratory disease which contributes to dyspnea. First, cessation of smoking is the only therapeutic intervention known to slow the accelerated decline in lung function in patients with COPD. Second, there is no currently available treatment which prolongs survival in patients with COPD.[1,2] The one exception to this statement is the use of supplemental oxygen in patients with hypoxemia who meet the criteria for prescribing oxygen established in the Nocturnal Oxygen Therapy Trial.[3]

Therefore, the major purpose for treating COPD, or any other chronic respiratory disease, should be: (1) to relieve symptoms, especially dyspnea; and (2) to enhance functional status. Improvement in dyspnea and/or daily function should lead to a better quality of life in affected individuals.

This chapter will examine available data on treating dyspnea as a major outcome variable. Specific consideration will be given to those clinical observations or trials which have used a valid, reliable, and sensitive instrument for measuring breathlessness. Most of these studies involve breathless patients with COPD. Only selected investigations involving healthy, asymptomatic individuals will be included in this review because information obtained in healthy subjects may have little, if any, direct application to patients experiencing dyspnea. It is likely, although unproven, that specific types of therapy for patients with COPD may be appropriate and useful for patients with other chronic respiratory disorders, e.g., cystic fibrosis or interstitial lung disease.

The benefits of breathing training techniques, especially body position, pursed-lips breathing, and diaphragmatic breathing, are described in Chapter 7, Coping and Self-Care Strategies.

II. Bronchodilator Medications

Bronchodilator medications are prescribed for relief of symptoms due to asthma, COPD, and cystic fibrosis. In 1984, Dull and Alexander[4] suggested that the acute response to an inhaled bronchodilator could be used to predict patients who will respond to treatment. If the FEV_1 increased by 15%, 25%, or more after an inhaled bronchodilator, then bronchodilator therapy was indicated; in contrast, if the FEV_1 improved by less than 15% or alternatively by less than 25%, then Dull and Alexander[4] proposed that bronchodilator medications may not be clinically useful based on the presumption that the disease was "non-reversible."

More recently, this approach has been reconsidered and reexamined for several reasons. First, every individual has some bronchomotor tone. An inhaled placebo *or* bronchodilator produces an increase of 7.7% to 12.3% in the baseline FEV_1 in a majority (greater than 95%) of asymptomatic, healthy individuals.[5-8] Second, the reproducibility of response to an inhaled bronchodilator is poor.[9,10] Guyatt et al.[10] reported that the correlation was only 0.17 ($p > 0.05$) for the percent change in FEV_1 after inhaled albuterol at 3 different visits in 24 patients with COPD. Third, the acute response to inhaled albuterol does not identify patients with COPD who are likely to benefit from either inhaled albuterol or sustained-release theophylline.[10]

Based on this information it is recommended that bronchodilator therapy be prescribed for all symptomatic patients with obstructive airway disease. Dyspnea (see Chapter 3) and lung function should be measured as baseline data and then repeated after a 2–4-week trial of a single bronchodilator medication. The results of subjective (dyspnea ratings) and/or objective (lung function) measurements should form the basis for assessing the benefits of a particular medication.

A. Beta-2 Adrenergic Agonist

Only two randomized controlled trials have examined the effect of an inhaled beta-2 adrenergic agonist on breathlessness in patients with COPD. Dullinger et al.[11] found that two puffs of metaproterenol given every 3 hours while awake for 1 week contributed to a significant improvement (+10%) in dyspnea on a 10 cm visual analogue scale (VAS). Guyatt and colleagues[12] reported similar findings in 19 patients with chronic airflow limitation who had less than a 25% increase in FEV_1 after inhalation of two puffs of albuterol. Breathlessness, as measured on a VAS at completion of a 6-minute walking test, improved with albuterol (Figure 1) as did the actual distance walked.[12] Lung function (FEV_1 and FVC) increased significantly after beta-2 adrenergic therapy in both investigations.[11,12]

Based on these two well-designed studies using appropriate methods for measuring breathlessness, both metaproterenol and albuterol relieve dyspnea despite modest, but significant, bronchodilatation.

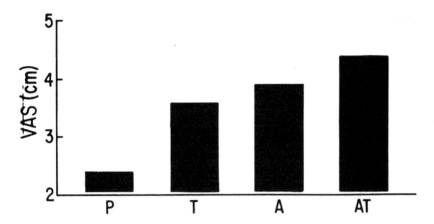

Figure 1: *Mean scores for dyspnea on a visual analogue scale (VAS) after a 6 minute walking test in 19 patients with COPD. P = placebo; T = theophylline; A = albuterol. Adapted from Guyatt GH, Townsend M, Pugsley SO, et al. Bronchodilators in chronic air-flow limitation: effects on airway function, exercise capacity, and quality of life. Am Rev Respir Dis 1987; 135:1069–1074, with permission.*

B. Anticholinergic Therapy

A paucity of data exists about the efficacy of inhaled anticholinergic therapy on the symptom of breathlessness. In a preliminary report on 32 patients with COPD, Hay et al.[13] observed improvement in ratings of dyspnea (Borg category scale) during cycle ergometry and a small increase of 160 mL in FEV_1 after inhalation of oxitropium in a double-blind, cross-over trial. Additional studies are necessary to evaluate the benefits of anticholinergic therapy for the sensation of dyspnea.

C. Theophylline

Seven studies have evaluated the efficacy of oral theophylline on ratings of dyspnea in COPD patients over at least a 1-week period[11,12,14–18] (Table 1). These investigations were all randomized, placebo-controlled, cross-over clinical trials. A majority of studies included only patients with either < 15%[16–18] or < 25%[10,11,15] improvement in FEV_1 after an inhaled bronchodilator in order to assess response in those patients with "non-reversible" airway obstruction.

Table 1. Effects of Theophylline on Lung Function and Ratings of Dyspnea in COPD

Study (reference #)	No. Subjects	Duration (weeks)	Change in FEV_1	Change in Dyspnea
Alexander[14]	40	4	+15%	"No improvement" (diary questionnaire)
Eaton[15]	14	1	+15%(low dose)* +12%(high dose)*	+25%(low dose) +15%(high dose) (VAS)
Mahler[16]	12	4	+10%	"Significant improvement" (p = 0.01 using BDI & TDI)*
Dullinger[11]	10	1	+12%	+6% (VAS)
Guyatt[12]	19	2	p = 0.002*	+50%* (VAS at end of 6 min walk test)
Chrystyn[17]	33	2	+13%*	+14%* (significant linear dose response using VAS)
Murciano[18]	60	8	+13%*	+25%* (VAS)

* = $p < 0.05$; VAS = visual analogue scale; BDI = baseline dyspnea index; TDI = transition dyspnea index.

In 1980, Alexander and colleagues[14] reported that FEV_1 increased by 15% with theophylline compared to placebo in 40 ambulatory patients with COPD. Although the authors noted "no improvement" in breathlessness on a diary questionnaire consisting of five descriptive responses, there was no information about the validity and reliability of the questionnaire.[14]

In 1982, Eaton et al.[15] studied 14 COPD patients over 1 week with low and high doses of theophylline. Although theophylline contributed to significant increases in FEV_1 (15% and 12% with low and high doses, respectively), the changes in dyspnea, as measured on a VAS, were +25% (low dose) and +15% (high dose) with theophylline. However, these improvements did not achieve statistical significance.

Three years later, Mahler et al.[16] found that clinical dyspnea ratings improved significantly after 4 weeks of sustained-release theophylline in 10 patients with non-reversible airflow obstruction (Figure 2). Although FEV_1 (+10%) and exercise capacity were greater with theophylline than with placebo, these changes were not significant.

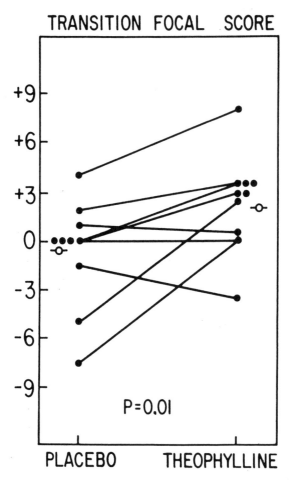

Figure 2: *Changes in dyspnea rating on the Transition Focal Score after 4 weeks of placebo and theophylline in 10 patients with "nonreversible" COPD. From Mahler DA, Matthay RA, Snyder PE, et al. Sustained-release theophylline reduces dyspnea in nonreversible obstructive airway disease. Am Rev Respir Dis 1985; 131:22–25, with permission.*

In 1986, Dullinger et al.[11] compared various treatment combinations, including placebo and theophylline, in 10 patients with COPD. Although both FEV_1 (+12%) and dyspnea (+6%) increased with theophylline, these trends were not statistically significant.

Guyatt and coworkers[12] also evaluated four different treatment periods, each of 2 weeks duration, in 19 patients with < 25% improvement in FEV_1 after inhaled albuterol. Theophylline led to significant improvements in FEV_1, 12-minute walking distance, and dyspnea ratings on the VAS (Figure 1).

In 1988, Chrystyn et al.[17] found a linear dose response for dyspnea (using VAS) in 33 COPD patients with increasing therapeutic levels of theophylline. In addition, there was a significant decrease in "trapped gas volume" and a corresponding increase in the 12-minute walking distance with high therapeutic levels of theophylline (Figure 3).

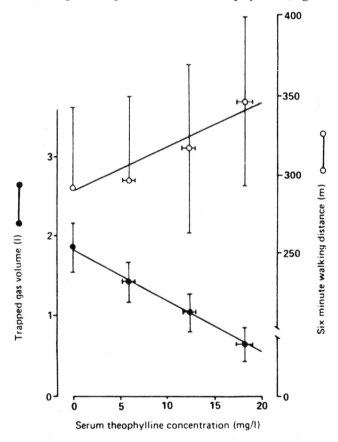

Figure 3: *Linear dose response for a decrease in trapped gas volume and 6 minute walking distance at 4 different serum theophylline concentrations in 33 patients with COPD. From Chrystyn H, Mulley BA, Peake MD. Dose response relation to oral theophylline in severe chronic obstructive airways disease. Br Med J 1988; 297:1506– 1510, with permission.*

Finally, Murciano et al.[18] examined 60 patients with "fixed airway obstruction" as defined by < 15% increase in FEV_1 after albuterol administration. These investigators found that after 2 months of theophylline, patients had significant improvements in dyspnea (+25% on the VAS), pulmonary gas exchange, FVC, FEV_1, and respiratory muscle performance.[18] Furthermore, there was a significant correlation ($r = 0.68$; $p < 0.001$) between the increase in respiratory muscle function and change in dyspnea with 2 months of theophylline therapy.

These overall results demonstrate a beneficial effect of theophylline on the sensation of breathlessness in patients with COPD with little evidence of airway "reversibility" by standard testing in the pulmonary function laboratory. Studies by Chrystyn et al.[17] and Murciano et al.[18] suggest that the improvement in dyspnea appears related, in part, to enhanced length-tension relationship of the diaphragm and/or an improvement in respiratory muscle function.

III. Environmental Conditions

A. Ambient Weather

Many patients with severe chronic respiratory disease describe increased breathlessness with extreme ambient air conditions. For example, hot, humid weather contributes to greater dyspnea possibly because irritants and pollutants become more concentrated in the ambient air. Also, cold and dry weather frequently leads to complaints of "difficulty" in breathing, presumably as a trigger for bronchoconstriction. Consequently, the "ideal" weather for breathing comfort appears to be clear skies with moderate temperature and humidity. Most symptomatic patients modify their activities based on the weather and "control" their indoor environment to avoid extreme conditions.

B. Air movement

Dyspneic patients frequently describe subjective improvement when sitting by an open window or when a portable fan blows air in their direction. In healthy, normal individuals cold air or liquid applied in the distribution of the trigeminal nerve decreases ventilation.[19,20] Schwartzstein et al.[21] reported that cold air directed against the cheek decreased breathlessness in six healthy individuals associated with the combined stimuli of hypercapnia and inspiratory resistance. These investigators hypothesized that stimulation of receptors on the face in the distribution of the trigeminal nerve provided afferent information to the sensory cortex which altered the perception of dyspnea.[21] However, there is little or no data on this phenomenon *in symptomatic patients.*

IV. Exercise

A. Aerobic Training

A number of controlled studies have described improvements in exercise capacity and skill performance due to exercise reconditioning programs in patients with COPD.[22–26] In addition, four of the reports describe a subjective reduction in dyspnea associated with exercise training compared to a control group.[22–24,26] However, a majority of these investigations did not use an appropriate instrument for measuring the sensation of breathlessness; rather, investigators asked patients to indicate improvement, no change, or deterioration in symptoms.

On the other hand, Strijbos and coworkers[26] examined Borg ratings of dyspnea during cycle ergometry in 45 patients with symptomatic COPD before and after 12 weeks of a pulmonary rehabilitation program consisting of relaxing exercises, breathing retraining, and exercise reconditioning. Patients were randomized into a treatment group (n = 30) and a control group (n = 15). At equivalent work loads, the treatment group showed a significant and marked decrease in dyspnea scores (p < 0.001), whereas the control group exhibited no significant change (Figure 4). Unfortunately, the investigators did not measure cardiorespiratory responses during exercise to evaluate potential mechanisms for relief of breathlessness.

A reduction in breathlessness with exercise training may be due to physiological and/or psychological factors. For example, selected studies report a decrease in exercise ventilation at comparable intensities of work after reconditioning.[25–28] Any decrease in the ventila-

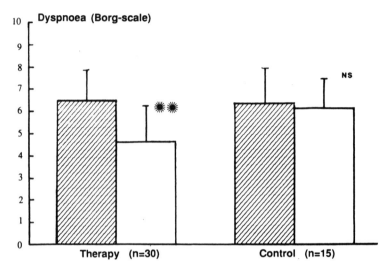

Figure 4: *Dyspnea scores on the Borg category scale at equivalent work loads on the cycle ergometer before and after a pulmonary rehabilitation program, including exercise reconditioning, in therapy and control groups. There was a significant decrease in scores for dyspnea after rehabilitation in the therapy group (p < 0.001). From Strijbos JH, Sluiter HJ, Postma DS, et al. Objective and subjective performance indicators in COPD. Eur Respir J 1989; 2:666–669, with permission.*

tory requirement for a given level of work might be expected to relieve dyspnea.[29] Furthermore, regular aerobic exercise may enhance a patient's tolerance of the distressful features of dyspnea, i.e., desensitization. Additional studies hopefully will examine the potential mechanisms for improvement in dyspnea with exercise reconditioning in patients with chronic respiratory disease. Meanwhile, aerobic training plays a key role in reconditioning programs with the concurrent goals of increasing functional capacity and decreasing the severity of breathlessness.

At the present time, there is no standardized approach for prescribing the intensity of exercise training for respiratory patients. A target heart rate and/or a target level of breathlessness can be used by the patient for estimating "how hard" to exercise; this information usually is obtained from results of a cardiopulmonary exercise test. The standard prescribed training intensity is 50% of peak exercise.[30] However, Ries and Archibald[31] have suggested that patients with COPD can train at levels approximating maximal exercise ventilation.

B. Continuous Positive Airway Pressure (CPAP)

O'Donnell and colleagues[32] have studied breathing pattern and respiratory sensation in response to expiratory resistance unloading in patients with severe COPD. Negative pressure applied at the mouth accentuated dynamic compression of airways downstream from the "choke point" or flow-limiting segment (Figure 5). With expiratory assistance, there were small but significant increases in f_R ($+2.3 \pm 0.7$ breaths/min) and $\dot{V}_E$ ($+1.5 \pm 0.6$ L/min) along with a highly significant ($p < 0.001$) increase in sense of breathing effort.[32]

Based on these findings, O'Donnell et al.[33] examined the effects of CPAP on respiratory sensation during submaximal exercise. These investigators hypothesized that administration of CPAP, which serves to unload the inspiratory muscles and attenuate dynamic compression on expiration, should improve breathlessness in patients with COPD. Although CPAP (4–5 cmH$_2$O) increased the sense of breathing effort in normal subjects, it resulted in a significant reduction ($p < 0.005$) in the effort of breathing in COPD patients. Partitioning of CPAP into continuous positive inspiratory pressure (CPIP) and continuous positive expiratory pressure (CPEP) components showed that CPIP facilitated breathing in patients with COPD, whereas CPEP led to inconsistent and insignificant results (Figure 6). These different responses suggest that CPAP improved respiratory sensation during exercise principally through its effect of unloading the inspiratory muscles.[33,34] In a subsequent study, O'Donnell et al.[35]

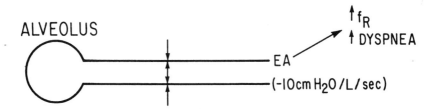

Figure 5: *Negative pressure (-10 cmH$_2$O/L/sec) applied at the mouth during expiration (expiratory assistance [EA]) accentuated dynamic compression of airways downstream from the "choke point" (opposing arrows) and led to increases in frequency of respiration (f_R) and minute ventilation along with an increase in dyspnea. Adapted from O'Donnell DE, Sanii R, Anthonisen NR, et al. Effect of dynamic airway compression on breathing pattern and respiratory sensation in severe chronic obstructive pulmonary disease. Am Rev Respir Dis 1987; 135:912–918.*

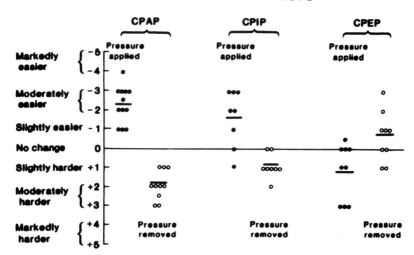

Figure 6: *Ratings of dyspnea on a category scale after application of continuous positive airway pressure (CPAP), continuous positive inspiratory pressure (CPIP), and continuous positive expiratory pressure (CPEP) during submaximal exercise in five patients with COPD. From O'Donnell DE, Sanii R, Giesbrecht G, et al. Effect of continuous positive airway pressure on respiratory sensation in patients with chronic obstructive pulmonary disease during submaximal exercise. Am Rev Respir Dis 1988; 138:1185–1191, with permission.*

found that CPAP also improved exercise endurance in COPD patients by alleviating exertional dyspnea.

C. Upper Extremity Training

Certain upper torso muscles, such as the pectoralis major and minor, latissimus dorsi, serratus anterior, and lower part of the trapezius, possess both a ribcage and a humeral-shoulder girdle attachment. This arrangement gives them both respiratory and postural functions depending on the fixation point from which they exert their pulling force. When these muscles are recruited to perform non-ventilatory work, particularly when the arms are unsupported, their participation in ventilation may be diminished. This observation may help explain the frequent onset of breathlessness in COPD patients when they perform seemingly trivial tasks with unsupported arms, such as brushing teeth, combing hair, etc.[36,37] Celli et al.[38] have reported that some patients with COPD experience an early onset of severe dyspnea associated with dyssynchronous thoracoabdominal breathing movements during arm exercise. This does not appear to be related to diaphragmatic fatigue.[38] Rather, patients with severe COPD may alter their breathing pattern when performing unsupported arm exercise by shifting a portion of the ventilatory burden away from the inspiratory muscles of the rib cage to the diaphragm and muscles of expiration.[39]

Although arm cranking has traditionally been an exercise used to train upper extremities, it actually bears little resemblance to the use of unsupported upper extremities in the activities of daily living. For these reasons, it is reasonable and appropriate that a pulmonary rehabilitation program include unsupported arm exercise. Ries et al.[40] reported that perceived breathlessness, as measured on a 10-point scale, improved after 6 weeks of upper extremity training for upper extremity performance tests and arm cycling.

Ideally, the training tasks should be relatively specific for activities of daily living. Generally, these exercises should include muscle groups of the elbow and the shoulder. The upper extremity training program should emphasize improvement in endurance as well as strength. A series of low-resistance, high-repetition exercises involving gravity resistance, with possible addition of light weights, should lead to increased endurance of arm and shoulder muscles. A typical training program might include a set of 10 repetitions of each exercise with light hand weights (1/2–2 kg). Daily exercise should include a series of five sets. Advancement to the next level can be made based on the training response and the ease/difficulty of performing the sets of arm exercises. Each exercise should be coordinated with respiration (entrainment); generally, patients are instructed to exhale with each repetitive effort.[40] In addition, progressive neuromuscular facilitation principles can be applied; diagonal (45°) combinations of muscle movements are used to strengthen weaker muscles by exercising functionally related muscles.[40]

V. Nutrition

The activities of eating, drinking, and breathing require coordination in order to prevent aspiration. When normal adults eat and drink, breathing becomes more irregular, and functional residual capacity decreases.[41,42] These mechanical changes may increase the work of breathing and contribute to dyspnea in some patients.

Nutritional status is an independent influence on the course of COPD.[43] Approximately one third of patients with COPD are significantly underweight.[44-46] Generally, diaphragm muscle mass decreases in proportion to body weight, and maximal respiratory pressures are reduced, at least in part, due to undernutrition.[47-49]

Based on this information, it is possible that nutritional repletion could enhance respiratory muscle strength and correspondingly reduce the experience of breathlessness. In one report, Wilson and colleagues[50] described oral nutritional repletion for 2 weeks in 6 patients with emphysema. Body weight increased by 6%, and maximal inspiratory and transdiaphragmatic pressures increased by similar percentages.[50] However, the increase in respiratory muscle strength could be attributable to learning or training effects as no control group was evaluated concurrently. On the other hand, Lewis et al.[51] examined 21 malnourished patients with COPD and divided them into a control group (n = 11), who consumed their usual diet, and a fed group (n = 10), who were given a high-calorie, high-protein supplement in addition to their usual diet. The authors found that the fed group consumed 174% ± 17% of the estimated basal energy expenditure, but they gained only 1 kg in body weight over the 8 weeks, and there was no change in respiratory muscle function.[51] Knowles et al.[52] observed a similar lack of improvement in respiratory muscle performance with dietary supplementation. More recently, Efthimiou et al.[53] performed a prospective, randomized, controlled trial to investigate the effect of supplementary oral nutrition over a 3-month period in poorly nourished patients with COPD. After 3 months of caloric repletion, there were significant increases in body weight, midarm muscle circumference, handgrip strength, and maximal inspiratory (PI_{MAX}) and expiratory (PE_{MAX}) pressures. In addition, improvement was observed in general well-being and breathlessness scores (1 to 5 scale and OCD), as well as 6-minute walking distance.[53]

Although increasing caloric intake in malnourished patients may be beneficial, absorption and metabolism of food results in an increase in carbon dioxide production ($\dot{V}CO_2$). Because $\dot{V}CO_2$ and ventilation are closely linked, ingestion of food may actually enhance ventilatory requirements and consequently affect dyspnea. Specifically, ingestion of carbohydrates causes a higher $\dot{V}CO_2$ per gram of food than do fats or protein.[54] Kwan and Mir[55] reported that 8 patients with chronic hypercapnic respiratory failure described an "improvement in general well-being" during 1-week periods of a low-carbohydrate diet along with a reduction in PCO_2 levels. In a randomized, double-blind study of 14 ambulatory patients with COPD, Angelillo et al.[56] found that a low carbohydrate diet (28% carbohydrate calories) resulted in significantly lower $\dot{V}CO_2$, respiratory quotient, and arterial PCO_2. In addition, Brown and co-workers[57-58] observed that a large carbohydrate load adversely affected exercise performance in patients with COPD. Although none of these investigations evaluated the symptom of breathlessness as an outcome variable, it is possible that a high-carbohydrate load may increase dyspnea. Therefore, a high-fat, low-carbohydrate diet may be beneficial in patients with severe airflow obstruction. However, further studies are needed before specific recommendations on nutrition can be made for relief of breathlessness.

VI. Oxygen

Hypoxemia is a potent ventilatory stimulus. By breathing oxygen, patients generally exhibit a decrease in ventilation (at rest and during exercise) and may experience less breathlessness.[59-63] Woodcock et al.[61] performed a double-blind, cross-over trial comparing the effects of air and oxygen on dyspnea and exercise tolerance in 10 patients with emphysema. The use of supplemental oxygen enabled these patients to walk farther and feel less breathless.[61] Davidson and associates[64] also found that oxygen significantly reduced breathlessness as well as the severity of arterial desaturation during exercise in 17 patients with COPD. One possible explanation for the beneficial effect of oxygen on the sensation of dyspnea is the reduction in the ventilatory response during exercise.

In addition, it has been suggested that supplemental oxygen may relieve dyspnea in selected patients who do not meet the standard criteria for oxygen prescription.[65,66] However, further guidelines are necessary for identifying and evaluating individual patients.

VII. Psychotropic Therapy

Psychotropic drugs, including benzodiazepines, opiates, and phenothiazines, have the potential to ameliorate the symptom of dyspnea. These agents might reduce breathlessness by depressing ventilation or by altering the integration and processing of the dyspnea "signal" in the central nervous system. Published studies involving psychotropic agents generally have demonstrated inconsistant results. Although opiates appear to offer the greatest potential benefit for relieving dyspnea, none of the psychotropic drugs should be routinely prescribed for treating dyspnea at the present time based on results of available studies. However, a single patient clinical trial may be appropriate in individuals who remain symptomatic despite otherwise "optimal" therapy.[67,68]

A. Benzodiazepines

Anxiety can be a major problem in patients with chronic respiratory disease and may directly contribute to the experience of dyspnea. Benzodiazepine drugs have the potential to relieve breathlessness by either their anxiolytic effect or possibly by an effect on the respiratory system. Their major physiological influence on respiration is depression of the hypoxic ventilatory response.[69,70] Several studies of different benzodiazepine agents have produced conflicting data (Table 2). In 1980, Mitchell-Heggs et al.[71] reported that 5 mg of diaz-

Table 2. Effects of Benzodiazepine Drugs on Ratings of Dyspnea in COPD

Study (reference #)	No. Subjects	Drug	Duration	Change in Dyspnea
Mitchell-Heggs[71]	4	diazepam	10–32 days	Improved (not measured)
Woodcock[72]	15	diazepam	14 days	No (VAS)
Eimer[73]	5	chlorazepate	14 days	No (OCD)
Man[74]	24	alprazolam	7 days	No (0–10 scale)
Green[75]	1	alprazolam	single dose	Yes (VAS)

VAS = visual analogue scale; OCD = oxygen-cost diagram.

epam given 5 times a day provided "a striking reduction in dys-pnoea" in 4 patients with predominant emphysema. However, there was no control group in this study and the authors did not measure breathlessness.[71] In a subsequent controlled study, Woodcock et al.[72] found that 25 mg of diazepam per day (given 3 times a day and at bedtime) had no effect on breathlessness and actually decreased exercise tolerance in 15 patients with emphysema. Eimer and colleagues[73] reported that 7.5 mg of clorazepate, another benzodiaz-epine drug, given at bedtime did not improve dyspnea in symptom-atic patients with COPD. Man and coworkers[74] performed a double-blind, cross-over trial of alprazolam, a benzodiazepine with a half-life of 10–12 hours. These investigators found that alprazolam was not effective in relieving exercise dyspnea over a 1-week period in 24 patients with COPD.[74] Finally, Green et al.[75] observed that a single dose of alprazolam reduced dyspnea in one anxious patient with COPD. However, this trial was neither blind nor controlled.

In summary, the results of available studies do not support the routine use of benzodiazepine drugs for treating dyspnea. However, anxiety can play a major role in an individual patient's difficulty in breathing, functional status, and quality of life. In such instances, a therapeutic trial may be considered as long as appropriate variables, e.g., anxiety, dyspnea, and exercise performance, are measured in order to evaluate the response.

B. Opiates

Opiates were used in the 19th century to relieve dyspnea, but their use was discontinued in the 1950s when it was recognized that res-piratory depression could develop.[76] In 1981, Woodcock et al.[77] dem-onstrated that a single dose of 1 mg/kg of oral dihydrocodeine de-creased breathlessness (Figure 7) and increased the walking distance on the treadmill in patients with COPD. Subsequently, Johnson et al.[78] evaluated the subacute administration of dihydrocodeine (15 mg up to 3 times a day) vs. placebo over a 1-week period in each of 18 patients with COPD who experienced severe breathlessness. With dihydro-codeine (average of 2.8 tablets per day), patients were less breathless (−17.8% on a daily VAS) and more mobile (+16.8% increase in pe-dometer distance). Furthermore, the authors reported that no adverse effects were encountered by the patients. On the other hand, higher doses of opiates appear to cause intolerable side effects. Woodcock et al.[79] administered 30 mg or 60 mg of dihydrocodeine 3 times a day

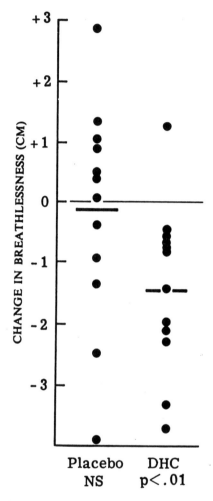

Figure 7: *Change in breathlessness on a visual analogue scale 45 minutes after placebo or dihydrocodeine (DHC) in 12 patients with COPD. A single dose of dihydrocodeine (1 mg/kg) significantly decreased breathlessness. From Woodcock AA, Gross ER, Gellert A, et al. Effects of dihydrocodeine, alcohol, and caffeine on breathlessness and exercise tolerance in patients with chronic obstructive long disease and normal blood gases. N Engl J Med 1981; 305:1611–1616, with permission.*

for 2 weeks in each of 16 patients with COPD. Although dyspnea on the OCD improved during the 30 mg period only, there was no change in the 6 minute walking distance with either dose. More importantly, substantial side effects developed, including nausea/

vomiting, constipation, and drowsiness, which caused considerable discomfort.[79] Rice et al.[80] found that codeine (30 mg 4 times a day) provided no improvement in breathlessness after a 1-month trial in patients with COPD, and that several subjects experienced mild narcotic withdrawal after discontinuation of codeine treatment.

Light et al.[81] recently evaluated the effects of a single dose of oral morphine solution (0.8 mg/kg) compared to placebo in 13 eucapnic patients with COPD. After ingestion of morphine, exercise performance increased significantly, and the Borg score for breathlessness at the highest equivalent workload was significantly lower with morphine compared to placebo (Figure 8). The improvement in exercise

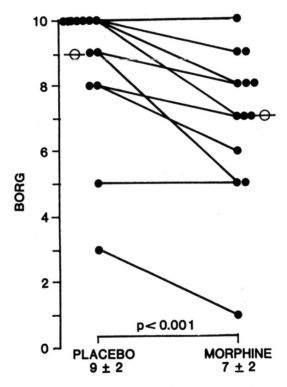

Figure 8: *Borg scores for dyspnea at the highest equivalent workload on the cycle ergometer 60 minutes after either placebo or oral morphine (0.8 mg/kg) in 13 patients with COPD. From Light RW, Muro JR, Sato RI, et al. Effects of oral morphine on breathlessness and exercise tolerance in patients with chronic obstructive pulmonary disease. Am Rev Respir Dis 1989; 139:126–133, with permission.*

tolerance was related to both a higher P_aCO_2 resulting in lowered ventilatory requirements and to a reduced perception of breathlessness for a given level of ventilation. Despite the documented benefits, Light et al.[81] conclude that substantial questions remain unanswered about the use of opiates in treating breathlessness in COPD and that routine administration should not be considered at the present time.

This recommendation appears warranted based on the concerns of safety, alteration in mental status, tolerance, and possible sleep related oxygen desaturation. On the other hand, use of oral or intravenous opiates is appropriate and justified for relieving the distressing experience of dyspnea during the terminal phase of care for patients with end-stage respiratory disease. In fact, the administration of opiates may provide a level of comfort and dignity otherwise not obtainable during the dying process.

C. Phenothiazines

Phenothiazines are another group of psychotropic agents which have been evaluated, to a limited extent, for the treatment of dyspnea. Woodcock et al.[72] reported that promethazine (25 mg 3 times a day and 50 mg at night) provided a modest reduction in breathlessness on a VAS during treadmill exercise and recovery compared to either placebo or diazepam. There was a concommitant 5% increase in the 12-minute walking distance with promethazine. In contrast, Rice and coworkers[80] reported that promethazine (25 mg 4 times a day) did not lead to any improvement in dyspnea or exercise capacity in 11 patients with COPD.

Based on the results of these two studies, there is no conclusive evidence that promethazine should be used routinely for treating breathlessness. However, it is possible that phenothiazine drugs may be helpful in selected individuals.

VIII. Respiratory Muscle Rest

Respiratory muscle weakness and fatigue may contribute to dyspnea, exercise limitation, and respiratory failure in patients with severe COPD.[82–84] Furthermore, it has been postulated that such patients may suffer from incipent or chronic respiratory muscle fatigue due to the increased work of breathing.[85,86] Therefore, resting the respiratory muscles potentially could improve respiratory muscle function and alleviate dyspnea.

Rochester and colleagues[87] found that assisted ventilation for short periods (about 20 minutes) resulted in significant reductions in electrical activity of the respiratory muscles, including the diaphragm, in 11 hypercapnic patients. Seven of these had COPD, and the intermittent assisted ventilation was reported to provide relief of dyspnea.[87] However, dyspnea was not quantified.

In a preliminary report, Braun and Marino[88] reported increases in both PI_{MAX} and PE_{MAX} and a reduction in P_aCO_2 in 14 COPD patients who received daily intermittent negative pressure ventilation using body wrap ventilation for 5 months. The authors also noted that subjects improved their overall functional status. However, a control group was not included for comparison, and it is possible that such improvements were related to enhanced medical care rather than to any specific effect of assisted ventilation.

Cropp and Dimarco[85] studied the effects of 3–6 hours of negative pressure ventilation for 3 consecutive days in 15 patients with stable COPD. Eight patients were in the experimental group and seven patients served as control subjects. After assisted ventilation, patients showed significant improvements in respiratory muscle strength (PI_{MAX} and PE_{MAX}) and endurance along with a mean decrease of 8 mmHg in P_aCO_2. The investigators noted that several experimental patients volunteered that their level of resting or exertional dyspnea had "improved substantially" after ventilator use, but they did not measure respiratory sensation.

Additional studies of external negative pressure ventilation in COPD patients have reported symptomatic improvement and/or subjective reductions in dyspnea based on comments by individual patients.[89–91] However, breathlessness was not directly measured in these clinical trials. Furthermore, patient acceptance and tolerance of external ventilation were variable, and physiological benefits are uncertain in randomized populations of patients with COPD.[90–91]

Recently, Martin[92] reported the preliminary results of a randomized trial of external negative pressure ventilation using a body wrap versus sham ventilatory muscle rest in 184 patients with COPD. Subjects used either the active treatment or sham for 8 hours per day during the daytime or nighttime. Baseline measures were obtained during hospitalization, including evaluation of supression of diaphragmatic electrical activity during external negative pressure ventilation. There was no improvement in exercise tolerance, PI_{MAX}, PE_{MAX}, arterial blood gases, dyspnea as measured on the oxygen cost diagram, or quality of life with ventilatory support compared to sham treatment.

In summary, *some* patients with COPD might experience less breathlessness during and/or as a result of external negative pressure ventilation.[85,87–91] Although there are theoretical benefits for "resting" the muscles of respiration, additional studies are needed to further evaluate the physiological effects of ventilatory muscle rest. Based on the results of present data, external negative pressure ventilation cannot be recommended routinely for relief of breathlessness in symptomatic patients.

IX. Respiratory Muscle Training

In 1976, Leith and Bradley[93] showed that ventilatory muscle strength and endurance specifically can be increased in normal individuals by appropriate muscle training programs. Consequently, sustained hyperpnea or inspiratory resistive training has been applied in patients with COPD. A majority of studies have evaluated resistive breathing training because the training devices are portable, and therefore, training can be performed by outpatients. In contrast, sustained hyperpnea requires more sophisticated equipment and patients need to perform training sessions in a clinic or hospital setting.

Various studies show conflicting results on the benefits of inspiratory muscle training[94–110] (Table 3). The difficulties in interpreting these results include: (1) a 4-week duration of training may be too short to elicit a training response (4 studies); (2) a randomized control group was not available for comparison (7 studies); and (3) a target for training stimulus intensity with appropriate feedback to the patient was not included (14 studies). Furthermore, Belman et al.[106,108] have emphasized that the pattern of breathing during training should be controlled and that a feedback signal of the resistive load should be provided in order to regulate the training intensity and to ensure an adequate training stimulus. Except for recent reports,[107–110] previous

Table 3. Results of Inspiratory Muscle Training in Patients with COPD

Study (reference #)	Duration (weeks)	Randomized Control Group	Respiratory Muscle Strength	Endurance	Dyspnea	Exercise
Andersen[94]	4	No	—	—	↓	—
Pardy[95]	8	Yes (n = 8)	—	—	—	↑
Pardy[96]	8	No	NC	—	—	NC
Bjerre-Jepsen[97]	6	Yes (n = 14)	—	—	—	NC
Sonne[98]	6	Yes (n = 3)	—	+13%	—	↑
Andersen[99]	12	No	—	—	↓	↑
Moreno[100]	8	No	+30%	+109%	↓	—
Ambrosino[101]	4	No	—	—	—	NC
Chen[102]	4	Yes (n = 6)	+6%	+59%	—	NC
Falk[103]	12	Yes (n = 15)	—	—	↓	↑
Madsen[104]	6	No	—	—	—	↓
McKeon[105]	6	Yes (n = 8)	NC	↑	—	NC
Belman[106]	6	No	NC	+50%	—	—
Larson[107]	8	Yes (n = 12)	+20%	+81%	—	↑
Belman[108]	5	Yes (n = 9)	+30%	+13%	—	—
Harver[109]	8	Yes (n = 9)	+37%	+10%	↓	—
Goldstein[110]	4	Yes (n = 6)	-2%	+174%	—	NC

NC = no change; a line indicates variable was not measured.

studies have neither quantified the effective stimulus load nor provided patients with feedback on the intensity of respiratory effort during respiratory muscle training.

Despite the variations and limitations of published studies, it is clear that COPD patients can increase respiratory muscle strength and/or endurance with appropriate frequency, intensity, and duration of training. In five studies, investigators have reported improvement in the symptom of dyspnea associated with respiratory muscle training.[94,99,100,103,109] However, there was no control group in three of these studies.[94,99,100] Only Harver and colleagues[109] used a valid, reliable, and sensitive instrument for assessing breathlessness; the remaining four reports included subjective assessment of dyspnea[94,100] or a four-question dyspnea scoring scale.[99,103]

Harver et al.[109] performed a randomized, placebo-controlled, parallel design trial of targeted inspiratory muscle training over an

8-week period. Patients in both groups exercised using an inspiratory resistance device (PFLEX, Healthscan, Upper Montclair, NJ) which was modified to give visual feedback on breath-to-breath changes related to inspiratory mouth pressure. Patients were instructed to inspire with a force sufficient to significantly deflect the needle (by deflating the sleeve in series with the resistor). Those in the experimental group trained at all six levels of inspiratory resistance (range, 5–35 cmH$_2$O/L/s), whereas patients in the control group trained at a constant, nominal level of resistance (about 5 cmH$_2$O/L/sec). This was accomplished by removing the one-way expiratory valve from the end of the PFLEX device. The experimental group trained at approximately 30% of PI$_{MAX}$ measured at functional residual capacity (FRC) and achieved a significant increase ($+37\%$ $\pm$ 35%) in PI$_{MAX}$ FRC as a function of training. More importantly, patients in the experimental group showed significant improvements in each of the three categories of the Transition Dyspnea Index as well as the focal dyspnea score (p $=$ 0.003) (Figure 9). Furthermore, the changes in PI$_{MAX}$ measured at residual volume and MVV were significantly correlated with the magnitude of task and magnitude of effort affecting breathlessness.[109]

Based on the collective results of published studies, inspiratory muscle training should not be prescribed routinely for *all* breathless patients with COPD. It is likely that patients with diminished respiratory muscle strength without severe hyperinflation may benefit from inspiratory muscle training. In addition, a high level of motivation by the symptomatic patient appears to be very important for performing and continuing such exercise. At the present time, a trial of inspiratory muscle training should be considered if: (1) the patient remains troubled by dyspnea, i.e., breathlessness interferes with daily activities, despite bronchodilator therapy and a regular aerobic exercise program; and (2) the measured PI$_{MAX}$ FRC is decreased compared to the predicted age-related valve.

Additional studies are necessary to identify characteristics of patients who will benefit from respiratory muscle training. Recommended guidelines for respiratory muscle training are listed in Table 4. Although commercially available training devices are available, it is important to quantify the training intensity, e.g., threshold loading, and to control the frequency and/or pattern of breathing during training. A trial of 6 to 8 weeks may be necessary in order to achieve a training response.

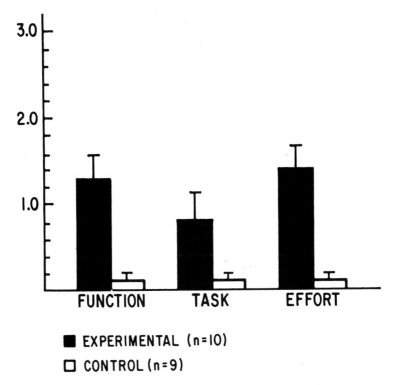

Figure 9: *Mean scores for each category of the Transition Dyspnea Index for experimental (closed bars) and control (open bars) subjects after 2 months of targeted inspiratory muscle training in patients with COPD. There was a significant improvement in each category of the dyspnea scores in the experimental group. From Harver A, Mahler DA, Daubenspeck JA. Targeted inspiratory muscle training improves respiratory muscle function and reduces dyspnea in patients with chronic obstructive pulmonary disease. Ann Intern Med 1989; 111:117–124, with permission.*

Table 4. Guidelines for Inspiratory Muscle Training

1. Frequency—at least 4–5 days/week
2. Intensity—25%–35% of maximal inspiratory mouth pressure (PI_{MAX}) measured at functional residual capacity (FRC).
3. Duration—two 15-minute sessions or one 30-minute session per day. If this cannot be achieved, the intensity can be reduced.

X. Summary

There are at least nine different general approaches or strategies for treating dyspnea in patients with COPD. These include: breathing training (pursed-lips, diaphragmatic breathing, and leaning forward position); bronchodilators; control of environmental conditions; exercise training; nutritional manipulations; oxygen therapy; psychotropic therapy; respiratory muscle rest; and respiratory muscle training. In addition, many of these treatment options may be applicable to other chronic respiratory diseases as well.

There is no established rank order for initiating these various therapeutic strategies in an individual patient. In general, one or more bronchodilators are prescribed as the initial approach for treating symptomatic patients with COPD. Depending on the impact of the disease, the physician or health-care provider should inform/ educate the patient concerning breathing training techniques in hopes to minimize the symptom of breathlessness. Although the patient usually learns about control of environmental conditions by day-to-day life experiences, this information should also be discussed with the patient in order to explain and clarify the importance of "controlling" the environment as much as possible. Based on the severity of physiological impairment, the physician certainly needs to measure the PaO_2 at rest and possibly during exercise to determine the need for supplemental oxygen.

Exercise training or reconditioning is often prescribed for patients who continue to be "limited" by breathlessness despite appropriate use of the aforementioned treatment options. Specific guidelines for exercise frequency, intensity, and duration ideally should be based on results of cardiopulmonary exercise testing. Exercise reconditioning may be done at a patient's home on an individual basis or may be part of a more organized pulmonary rehabilitation program.

Additional treatment options may be tried if the patient continues to experience dyspnea. However, precise selection criteria and specific directions for nutritional manipulations, respiratory muscle rest, and respiratory muscle training need to be established before these strategies can be routinely prescribed. In addition, it is possible, although unproven, that a combined approach of respiratory muscle training followed by respiratory muscle rest may provide optimal enhancement of respiratory muscle function and alleviate breathlessness. Opiates should be reserved, at the present time, for symptomatic care of end-stage chronic respiratory disease.

References

1. Burrows B, Earle RH. Course and prognosis of chronic obstructive lung disease. N Engl J Med 1969; 280:397-404.
2. Emirgil C, Sobol BJ. Long-term course of chronic obstructive pulmonary disease. Am J Med 1971; 51:504-512.
3. Nocturnal Oxygen Therapy Trial Group. Continuous or nocturnal oxygen therapy in hypoxemic obstructive lung disease. Ann Intern Med 1980; 93:391-398.
4. Dull WL, Alexander MR. Theophylline in stable chronic airflow obstruction: a reappraisal. Arch Intern Med 1984; 144:2399-2401.
5. Watanobe S, Renzetti AD, Begin R, et al. Airway responsiveness to a bronchodilator aerosol. Am Rev Respir Dis 1974; 109:530-537.
6. Lorber DB, Kaltenborn W, Burrows B. Responses to isoproterenol in a general population sample. Am Rev Respir Dis 1978; 118:855-861.
7. Sourk RL, Nugent KM. Bronchodilator testing: confidence intervals derived from placebo inhalations. Am Rev Respir Dis 1983; 128:153-157.
8. Dales RE, Spitzer WO, Tousignant P, et al. Clinical interpretation of airway response to a bronchodilator: epidemiologic considerations. Am Rev Respir Dis 1988; 138:317-320.
9. Anthonisen NR, Wright EC, IPPB Trial Group. Bronchodilator response in chronic obstructive pulmonary disease. Am Rev Respir Dis 1986; 133:814-819.
10. Guyatt GH, Townsend M, Nogradi S, et al. Acute response to bronchodilator: an imperfect guide for bronchodilator therapy in chronic airflow limitation. Arch Intern Med 1988; 148:1949-1952.
11. Dullinger D, Kronenberg R, Niewoehner DE. Efficacy of inhaled metaproterenol and orally-administered theophylline in patients with chronic airflow obstruction. Chest 1986; 89:171-173.
12. Guyatt GH, Townsend M, Pugsley SO, et al. Bronchodilators in chronic air-flow limitation: Effects on airway function, exercise capacity, and quality of life. Am Rev Respir Dis 1987; 135:1069-1074.
13. Hay JG, Stone P, Carter J, et al. Breathlessness and exercise performance in COPD - the effect of anti-cholinergic therapy. Am Rev Respir Dis 1989; 139(suppl):A333.
14. Alexander MR, Dull WL, Kasik JE. Treatment of chronic obstructive pulmonary disease with orally administered theophylline: a double-blind, controlled study. JAMA 1980; 244:2286-2290.
15. Eaton ML, MacDonald FM, Church TR, et al. Effects of theophylline on breathlessness and exercise tolerance in patients with chronic airflow obstruction. Chest 1982; 82:538-542.
16. Mahler DA, Matthay RA, Snyder PE, et al. Sustained-release theophylline reduces dyspnea in nonreversible obstructive airway disease. Am Rev Respir Dis 1985; 131:22-25.

17. Chrystyn H, Mulley BA, Peake MD. Dose response relation to oral theophylline in severe chronic obstructive airways disease. Br Med J 1988; 297:1506-1510.
18. Murciano D, Auclair MH, Pariente R, et al. A randomized, controlled trial of theophylline in patients with severe chronic obstructive pulmonary disease. N Engl J Med 1989; 320:1521-1525.
19. McBride B, Whitelaw WA. A physiological stimulus to upper airway receptors in humans. J Appl Physiol 1981; 51:1189-1197.
20. Burgess KR, Whitelaw WA. Reducing ventilatory responses to carbon dioxide by breathing air. Am Rev Respir Dis 1984; 129:687-690.
21. Schwartzstein RM, Lahive K, Pope A, et al. Cold facial stimulation reduces breathlessness in normal subjects. Am Rev Respir Dis 1987; 136: 58-61.
22. Cockcroft AE, Saunders MT, Berry G. Randomized controlled trial of rehabilitation in chronic respiratory disability. Thorax 1981; 36:200-203.
23. McGavin CR, Gupta SP, Lloyd EL, et al. Physical rehabilitation of chronic bronchitis: results of a controlled trial of exercise in the home. Thorax 1977; 32:307-311.
24. Sinclair DJM, Ingram CG. Controlled trial of supervised exercise training in chronic bronchitis. Br Med J 1980; 280:519-521.
25. Chester EH, Belman MJ, Bahler RC, et al. Multi-disciplinary treatment of chronic pulmonary insufficiency. 3. The effect of physical training on cardiopulmonary performance in patients with chronic obstructive pulmonary disease. Chest 1977; 72:695-702.
26. Strijbos JH, Sluiter HJ, Postma DS, et al. Objective and subjective performance indicators in COPD. Eur Respir J 1989; 2:666-669.
27. Pierce AK, Taylor HF, Archer RF, et al. Responses to exercise training in patients with emphysema. Arch Intern Med 1964; 113:28-36.
28. Christie D. Physical training in chronic obstructive lung disease. Br Med J 1968; 2:150-151.
29. Casaburi R, Wasserman K. Exercise training in pulmonary rehabilitation (editorial). N Engl J Med 1986; 314:1509-1511.
30. American College of Sports Medicine Position Stand on the Recommended Quantity and Quality of Exercise for Developing and Maintaining Cardiorespiratory and Muscular Fitness in Healthy Adults. Med Sci Sports Exerc 1990; 22:265-274.
31. Ries AL, Archibald CJ. Endurance exercise training at maximal targets in patients with COPD. J Cardiopulm Rehab 1987; 7:594-601.
32. O'Donnell DE, Sanii R, Anthonisen NR, et al. Effect of dynamic airway compression on breathing pattern and respiratory sensation in severe chronic obstructive pulmonary disease. Am Rev Respir Dis 1987; 135: 912-918.
33. O'Donnell DE, Sanii R, Giesbrecht G, et al. Effect of continuous positive airway pressure on respiratory sensation in patients with chronic obstructive pulmonary disease during submaximal exercise. Am Rev Respir Dis 1988; 138:1185-1191.
34. Petrof B, Calderini E, Gottfried SB. Continuous positive airway pressure

(CPAP) improves respiratory muscle performance and dyspnea during exercise in severe chronic obstructive pulmonary disease (COPD). Am Rev Respir Dis 1989; 139(suppl):A343.

35. O'Donnell DE, Sanii R, Younes M. Improvement in exercise endurance in patients with chronic airflow limitation using continuous positive airway pressure. Am Rev Respir Dis 1988; 138:1510-1514.

36. Tangri S, Woolf CR. The breathing pattern in chronic obstructive lung disease during performance of some common daily activities. Chest 1973; 63:126-127.

37. Celli BR. Arm exercise and ventilation (editorial). Chest 1988; 93:673-674.

38. Celli BR, Rassulo J, Make BJ. Dyssynchronous breathing during arm but not leg exercise in patients with chronic airflow obstruction. N Engl J Med 1986; 314:1485-1490.

39. Criner GJ, Celli BR. Effect of unsupported arm exercise on ventilatory muscle recruitment in patients with severe chronic airflow obstruction. Am Rev Respir Dis 1988; 138:856-861.

40. Ries AL, Ellis B, Hawkins RW. Upper extremity exercise training in chronic obstructive pulmonary disease. Chest 1988; 93:688-692.

41. Smith J, Wolkovc N, Colacone A, et al. Coordination of eating, drinking and breathing in adults. Chest 1989; 96:578-582.

42. Gilroy RJ Jr, Lavietes MH, Loring SH, et al. Respiratory mechanical effects of abdominal distension. J Appl Physiol 1985; 58:1997-2003.

43. Wilson DO, Rogers RM, Wright EC, et al. Body weight in chronic obstructive pulmonary disease. Am Rev Respir Dis 1989; 139:1435-1438.

44. Openbrier R, Irwin MM, Rogers RM, et al. Nutritional status and lung function in patients with emphysema and chronic bronchitis. Chest 1983; 83:17-22.

45. Hunter AM, Curey MA, Larsh MW. The nutritional status of patients with chronic obstructive pulmonary disease. Am Rev Respir Dis 1985; 124:376-381.

46. Rochester DF. Body weight and respiratory muscle function in chronic obstructive pulmonary disease (editorial). Am Rev Respir Dis 1986; 134: 646-648.

47. Arora NS, Rochester DF. Effect of body weight and muscularity on human diaphragm muscle mass, thickness, and area. J Appl Physiol 1982; 52:64-70.

48. Thurlbeck WM. Diaphragm and body weight in emphysema. Thorax 1978; 33:483-487.

49. Arora NS, Rochester DF. Respiratory muscle strength and maximal voluntary ventilation in undernourished patients. Am Rev Respir Dis 1982; 126:5-8.

50. Wilson DO, Rogers RM, Sanders MH, et al. Nutritional intervention in malnourished patients with emphysema. Am Rev Respir Dis 1986; 134: 672-677.

51. Lewis MI, Belman MJ, Dorr-Uyemura L. Nutritional supplementation in ambulatory patients with chronic obstructive pulmonary disease. Am Rev Respir Dis 1987; 135:1062-1068.

52. Knowles JB, Fairbarn MS, Wiggs BJ, et al. Dietary supplementation and respiratory muscle performance in patients with COPD. Chest 1988; 93:977-983.
53. Efthimiou J, Fleming J, Gomes C, et al. The effect of supplementary oral nutrition in poorly nourished patients with chronic obstructive pulmonary disease. Am Rev Respir Dis 1988; 137:1075-1082.
54. Saltzman HA, Salzano JV. Effects of carbohydrate metabolism upon respiratory gas exchance in normal men. J Appl Physiol 1971; 30:228-231.
55. Kwan R, Mir MA. Beneficial effects of dietary carbohydrate restriction in chronic cor pulmonale. Am J Med 1987; 82:751-758.
56. Angelillo VA, Sukhdarshan B, Durfee D, et al. Effects of low and high carbohydrate feedings in ambulatory patients with chronic obstructive pulmonary disease and chronic hypercapnia. Ann Intern Med 1985; 103:883-885.
57. Brown SE, Weiner S, Brown RA, et al. Exercise performance following a carbohydrate load in chronic airflow obstruction. J Appl Physiol 1985; 58:1340-1346.
58. Brown SE, Nagendran RC, McHugh JW, et al. Effects of a large carbohydrate load on walking performance in chronic air-flow obstruction. Am Rev Respir Dis 1985; 132:960-962.
59. Vyas MN, Banister EW, Morton JW, et al. Response to exercise in patients with chronic airway obstruction. II. Effects of breathing 40 percent oxygen. Am Rev Respir Dis 1971; 103:401-412.
60. Bradley BL, Garner AE, Billiu D, et al. Oxygen-assisted exercise in chronic obstructive lung disease: the effect on exercise capacity and arterial blood gas tensions. Am Rev Respir Dis 1978; 118:239-243.
61. Woodcock AA, Gross ER, Geddes DM. Oxygen relieves breathlessness in "pink puffers". Lancet 1981; i:907-909.
62. Swinburn CR, Wakefield JM, Jones PW. Relationship between ventilation and breathlessness during exercise in chronic obstructive airways disease is not altered by prevention of hypoxemia. Clin Sci 1984; 67:515-519.
63. Lane R, Cockcroft A, Adams L, et al. Arterial oxygen saturation and breathlessness in patients with chronic obstructive airways disease. Clin Sci 1987; 72:693-698.
64. Davidson AC, Leach R, George RJD, et al. Supplemental oxygen and exercise ability in chronic obstructive airways disease. Thorax 1988; 43:965-971.
65. Criner GJ, Celli BR. Ventilatory muscle recruitment in exercise with O_2 in obstructed patients with mild hypoxemia. J Appl Physiol 1987; 63:195-200.
66. Stulbarg MS, Dean NC, Himelman RB, et al. Oxygen (O_2) may improve dyspnea and endurance in COPD patients with only mild hypoxemia. Am Rev Respir Dis 1989; 139(suppl):A331.
67. Guyatt G, Sackett D, Taylor W, et al. Determining optimal therapy: randomized trials in individual patients. N Engl J Med 1986; 314:889-892.

68. Robin ED, Burke CM. Single-patient randomized clinical trial: opiates for intractable dyspnea. Chest 1986; 90:888-892.
69. Lakshminarayan S, Sahn SA, Hudson LD, et al. Effect of diazepam on ventilatory responses. Clin Pharmacol Ther 1976; 20:178-183.
70. Rao S, Sherbaniuk RW, Prasad K, et al. Cardiopulmonary effects of diazepam. Clin Pharmacol Ther 1972; 14:182-189.
71. Mitchell-Heggs P, Murphy K, Minty K, et al. Diazepam in the treatment of dyspnea in the "pink puffer" syndrome. Q J Med 1980; 49:9-20.
72. Woodcock AA, Gross ER, Geddes DM. Drug treatment of breathlessness: contrasting effects of diazepam and promethazine in pink puffers. Br Med J 1981; 283:343-346.
73. Eimer M, Cable T, Gal P, et al. Effects of clorazepate on breathlessness and exercise tolerance in patients with chronic airflow obstruction. J Fam Pract 1985; 21:359-362.
74. Man GCW, Hsu K, Sproule BJ. Effect of alprazolam on exercise and dyspnea in patients with chronic obstructive pulmonary disease. Chest 1986; 90:832-836.
75. Green JG, Pucino F, Carlson JD, et al. Effects of alprazolam on respiratory drive, anxiety, and dyspnea in chronic airflow obstruction: a case study. Pharmacotherapy 1989; 9:34-38.
76. Wilson RH, Hoseth W, Dempsey ME. Respiratory acidosis. I. Effects of decreasing respiratory minute volume in patients with severe chronic pulmonary emphysema, with specific reference to oxygen, morphine, and barbiturates. Am J Med 1954; 17:464-470.
77. Woodcock AA, Gross ER, Gellert A, et al. Effects of dihydrocodeine, alcohol, and caffeine on breathlessness and exercise tolerance in patients with chronic obstructive lung disease and normal blood gases. N Engl J Med 1981; 305:1611-1616.
78. Johnson MA, Woodcock AA, Geddes DM. Dihydrocodeine for breathlessness in "pink puffers." Br Med J 1983; 286:675-677.
79. Woodcock AA, Johnson MA, Geddes DM. Breathlessness, alcohol, and opiates (letter to the editor). N Engl J Med 1982; 306:1363-1364.
80. Rice KL, Kronenberg RS, Hedemark LL, et al. Effects of chronic administration of codeine and promethazine on breathlessness and exercise tolerance in patients with chronic airflow obstruction. Br J Dis Chest 1987; 81:287-292.
81. Light RW, Muro JR, Sato RI, et al. Effects of oral morphine on breathlessness and exercise tolerance in patients with chronic obstructive pulmonary disease. Am Rev Respir Dis 1989; 139:126-133.
82. Roussos C. Function and fatigue of respiratory muscles. Chest 1985; 88:1245-1305.
83. Belman MJ, Sieck GC. The ventilatory muscles: fatigue, endurance, and training. Chest 1982; 82:761-766.
84. Cohen CA, Zagelbaum G, Gross D, et al. Clinical manifestations of inspiratory muscle fatigue. Am J Med 1982; 73:308-316.
85. Cropp A, Dimarco AF. Effects of intermittent negative pressure ventilation on respiratory muscle function in patients with severe chronic

obstructive pulmonary disease. Am Rev Respir Dis 1987; 135:1056-1061.
86. Rochester DF. Does respiratory muscle rest relieve fatigue or incipient fatigue? (editorial). Am Rev Respir Dis 1988; 138:516-517.
87. Rochester DF, Braun NMT, Lane S. Diaphragmatic energy expenditure in chronic respiratory failure: the effect of assisted ventilation with body respirators. Am J Med 1977; 63:223-232.
88. Braun NMT, Marino WD. Effect of daily intermittent rest of respiratory muscles in patients with severe chronic airflow limitation (CAL). Chest 1984; 85(suppl):59S.
89. Gutierrez M, Beroiza T, Contreras G, et al. Weekly curiass ventilation improves blood gases and inspiratory muscle strength in patients with chronic air-flow limitation and hypercapnia. Am Rev Respir Dis 1988; 138:617-623.
90. Zibrak JD, Hill NS, Federman EC, et al. Evaluation of intermittent long-term negative-pressure ventilation in patients with severe chronic obstructive pulmonary disease. Am Rev Respir Dis 1988; 138:1515-1518.
91. Celli B, Lee H, Criner G, et al. Controlled trial of external negative pressure ventilation in patients with severe chronic airflow obstruction. Am Rev Respir Dis 1989; 140:1251-1256.
92. Martin JG. Clinical intervention in chronic respiratory failure. Chest 1990; 97(suppl):105S-109S.
93. Leith DE, Bradley M. Ventilatory muscle strength and endurance training. J Appl Physiol 1976; 41:508-516.
94. Andersen JB, Dragsted L, Kann T, et al. Resistive breathing training in severe chronic obstructive pulmonary disease: a pilot study. Scand J Respir Dis 1979; 60:151-156.
95. Pardy RL, Rivington RN, Despas PJ, et al. Inspiratory muscle training compared with physiotherapy in patients with chronic airflow limitation. Am Rev Respir Dis 1981; 123:421-425.
96. Pardy RL, Rivington RN, Despas PJ, et al. The effects of inspiratory muscle training on exercise performance in chronic airflow limitation. Am Rev Respir Dis 1981; 123:426-433.
97. Bjerre-Jepsen K, Secher NH, Kok-Jensen A. Inspiratory resistance training in severe chronic pulmonary disease. Eur J Respir Dis 1981; 62:405-411.
98. Sonne LJ, Davis JA. Increased exercise performance in patients with severe COPD following inspiratory resistive training. Chest 1982; 81:436-439.
99. Andersen JB, Falk P. Clinical experience with inspiratory resistive breathing training. Int Rehabil Med 1984; 6:183-185.
100. Moreno R, Moreno R, Guigliano C, et al. Entrenamiento muscular inspiratorio en pacientes con limitacion chronica del flujo aereo. Rev Med Chile 1983; 111:647-653.
101. Ambrosino N, Paggiaro PL, Roselli MG, et al. Failure of resistive breathing training to improve pulmonary function tests in patients with chronic obstructive pulmonary disease. Respiration 1984; 45:455-459.

102. Chen HI, Dukes R, Martin BJ, Inspiratory muscle training in patients with chronic obstructive pulmonary disease. Am Rev Respir Dis 1985; 131:251-255.
103. Falk P, Eriksen AM, Kolliker K, et al. Relieving dyspnea with an inexpensive and simple method in patients with severe chronic airflow limitation. Eur J Respir Dis 1985; 66:181-186.
104. Madsen F, Secher NH, Kay L, et al. Inspiratory resistance versus general physical training in patients with chronic obstructive pulmonary disease. Eur J Respir Dis 1985; 67:167-176.
105. McKeon JL, Turner J, Kelly C, et al. The effect of inspiratory resistive training on exercise capacity in optimally treated patients with severe chronic airflow limitation. Aust N Z J Med 1986; 16:648-652.
106. Belman MJ, Thomas SG, Lewis MI. Resistive breathing training in patients with chronic obstructive pulmonary disease. Chest 1986; 90:662-669.
107. Larson JL, Kim MJ, Sharp JT, et al. Inspiratory muscle training with a pressure threshold breathing device in patients with chronic obstructive pulmonary disease. Am Rev Respir Dis 1988; 138:689-696.
108. Belman MJ, Shadmehr R. Targeted resistive ventilatory muscle training in chronic obstructive pulmonary disease. J Appl Physiol 1988; 65:2726-2735.
109. Harver A, Mahler DA, Daubenspeck JA. Targeted inspiratory muscle training improves respiratory muscle function and reduces dyspnea in patients with chronic obstructive pulmonary disease. Ann Intern Med 1989; 111:117-124.
110. Goldstein R, DeRosie J, Long S, et al. Applicability of a threshold loading device for inspiratory muscle testing and training in patients with COPD. Chest 1989; 96:564-571.

Index